diabetes
BREAKTHROUGHS
2011

diabetes
BREAKTHROUGHS
2011

Proven Approaches
to Take Back Your Life

FROM THE EDITORS OF **Prevention**

RODALE

Prevention is a registered trademark of Rodale Inc.

Printed in the United States of America
Rodale Inc. makes every effort to use acid-free ♾, recycled paper ♻.

Photo credits are on page 355.
Book design by Chalkley Calderwood

ISBN-13: 978–1–60529–170–3

2   4   6   8   10   9   7   5   3   1   hardcover

For more of our products visit **prevention.com** or call 800-848-4735

CONTENTS

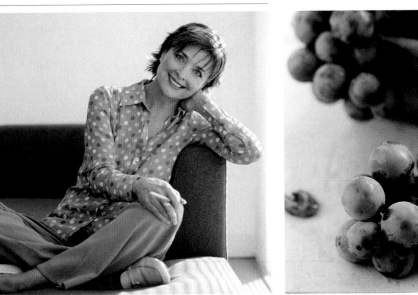

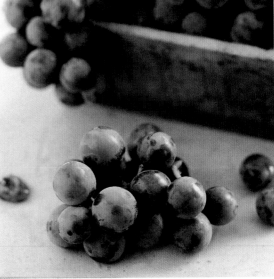

PART

1
TAKE CONTROL

PART

2
EAT RIGHT

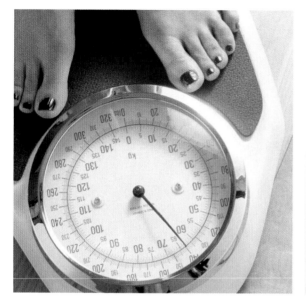

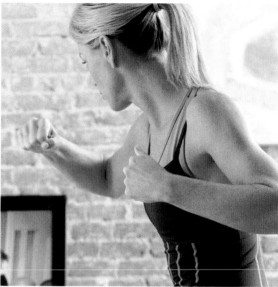

PART

3

LOSE WEIGHT

PART

4

MOVE IT

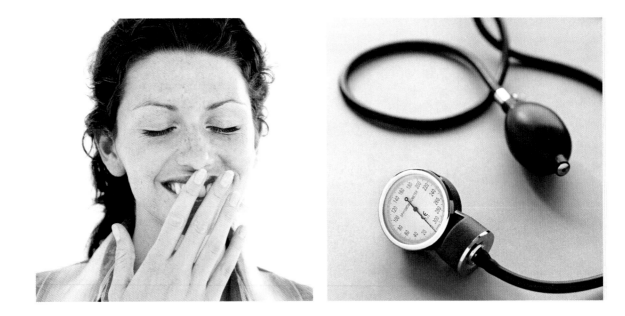

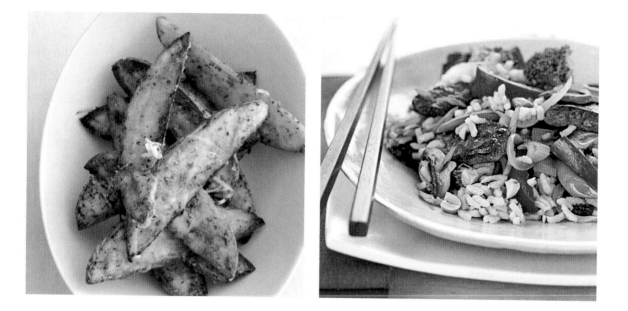

PART

7

DIABETES COOKBOOK

INTRODUCTION

Whether you've been diagnosed with prediabetes or diabetes—or someone you love has—your life has been dramatically changed. Finding out that you have a condition like diabetes can be shocking, unsettling, and worrying. But it can also be empowering.

Now you know what you have to do: Take control of your blood sugar. And the book you're holding in your hands will explain how to do that.

Let's begin at the beginning. Part 1 will help you "Take Control." You'll learn why it's so important to get your blood sugar in check, and then how to do so. You'll also discover other critical information about medications.

In Part 2, you'll find out how to "Eat Right." Nutrition is very important for people with diabetes, and adjusting your diet might help you avoid having to take any medication for your diabetes at all. From shopping to cooking to eating smart, this section covers it all.

Part 3 explains why it's so important to "Lose Weight." It's shocking that 9 out of 10 people who have been diagnosed with diabetes are overweight. Here you'll find simple solutions to taking off the pounds, including that so-very-hard-to-lose belly fat.

You'll "Move It" more after reading Part 4. After reading in Chapter 17 about the top 10 reasons you should "Move More," you'll find some simple ways to incorporate exercise into your life, such as easy walking plans and workouts you can do right in your living room—no need to step foot in a gym.

In Part 5, you'll discover the connection between mind and body in "Mind Matters." Like so many things that ail the body, diabetes has a strong mental connection. Stress certainly makes diabetes worse, so stressing less can help. You'll also find out how to boost your willpower, brainpower, and even your happiness.

Part 6 discusses the many complications of diabetes, so this section will help you "Avoid Complications." Here you'll learn how to prevent some of the most common diabetes-related ills, including erectile dysfunction, high blood pressure, and even cancer.

You'll get cooking tips in Part 7 with our "Diabetes Cookbook." We've gathered this year's 100 best recipes for people with diabetes. Some of our favorites are Sweet Lemon-Ricotta Brunch Blintzes (see page 240), Scrambled Egg "Pizza" (see page 236), "Fried" Zucchini Sticks with Marinara Sauce (see page 246), Instant Garden Salad (see page 256), French Onion Soup (see page 267), Old-Fashioned Creamed Spinach (see page 281), Spinach Lasagna (see page 290), Double Roasted Chicken (see page 301), Spicy Rubbed Pork Tenderloin with Edamame Succotash (see page 322), Mustard- and Brown Sugar-Rubbed Salmon (see page 340), and Rich Chocolate Torte (see page 349). We hope you love them, too.

Getting a diabetes diagnosis may have thrown you a curveball. But with this information at your fingertips, you can take control—and take back your life.

1

TAKE

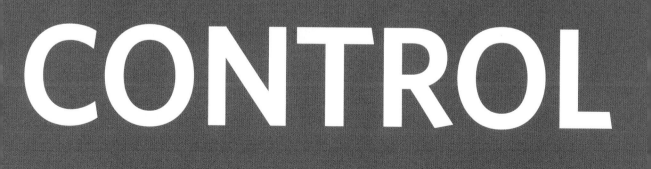

CONTROL

to help you better manage diabetes.

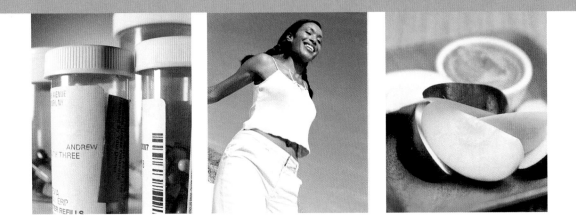

DIAGNOSTIC
Medical Breakthroughs

Information is power, and knowledge offers comfort. After you receive a diagnosis like diabetes, gathering information can give you a sense of control. **Here is the latest research about diabetes diagnostics to help you take charge of your health.**

REACH YOUR HEALTH GOALS

Here are two simple, proven ways to help attain a health goal.

Ask for an exercise Rx: Inactive people given prescriptions from a doctor got more activity (about 18 minutes a week) than those who didn't, according to a new Spanish study. Your doctor may be an especially helpful coach if you have a condition (such as diabetes) affecting your ability to exercise. Or ask for a referral to a certified fitness professional.

Set up regular e-mail reminders: In a Kaiser Permanente study, people who received personalized weekly e-mails about nutritious snack ideas or making time for workouts adopted significantly healthier habits than those who didn't. Reap similar benefits by setting your own daily calendar messages. Choose small goals that are achievable and practical, such as "11:00 a.m.: Take a walk for 10 minutes"; "3:30 p.m.: Eat an apple and peanut butter."

SCHEDULE A CHECKUP

A regular dental checkup can actually be lifesaving. Your dentist is the health provider who is most likely to detect bleeding gums, which can be a sign of more than 20 conditions, including diabetes, hormonal imbalances, cancer, and a vitamin deficiency, according to Chicago-area dentist Ronald Schefdore, DMD.

Dentists can also prescribe home screening tests (such as ones used to gauge systemic inflammation) for many diseases—often at a fraction of the cost of a hospital blood test, he points out.

TURN OFF THE TUBE

It's a startling fact that, on average, Americans watch 151 hours of TV per month. That's 37.75 hours a week—practically a full-time job.

All of this screen time comes at a high price. Watching just 60 hours of TV per month is associated with a 23 percent higher risk of obesity and a 14 percent increased risk of diabetes.

Experts say that for ideal health, the recommended number of hours of TV per month is far lower: only 30 hours.

The percentage of people who say online health records would prevent medical errors, according to the Markle Foundation:

65

GET YOUR MEDS BY MAIL ORDER

When you fill your prescription through a reputable mail order pharmacy, you're more likely to take it as directed and gain maximum benefit from the drug, according to a new study by Emily Cox, PhD, for the drug-benefit provider Express Scripts.

Among people taking meds for diabetes, hypertension, and high cholesterol, Dr. Cox found that up to 82 percent who use home delivery swallow their pills on time and as prescribed, compared with 71 percent of people who fill their scripts at a retail pharmacy.

One reason: You can fill 3 months of a medication at a time with mail order pharmacies, which means fewer chances to forget refills and miss doses.

Don't Let Your Meds Mess with Your Blood Sugar

Certain drugs can worsen diabetes by interfering with insulin or blood sugar levels, says Anne L. Peters, MD, director of the clinical diabetes programs at the University of Southern California in Los Angeles. Ask your doctor about possible safer alternatives.

The Drug	*The Risk*	*The Alternatives*
OTC decongestants (original Sudafed, Advil Allergy Sinus)	Pseudoephedrine, an active ingredient, spurs adrenaline (the fight-or-flight response), causing blood sugar to rise.	Pseudoephedrine-free decongestants (Sudafed PE) or nondrug remedies for stuffiness, such as neti pots
Steroids (cortisone, prednisone)	These anti-inflammatories can boost blood sugar levels by making your body less sensitive to insulin.	NSAIDs (Advil, Relafen)
Diuretics (Lasix, Bumex)	Used for high blood pressure, diuretics can deplete potassium, interfering with the pancreas's ability to secrete insulin.	ACE inhibitors (Zestril, Vasotec); angiotensin II receptor blockers (Avapro, Cozaar)
Beta-blockers (Inderal, Corgard)	These blood pressure regulators increase insulin resistance.	Angiotensin II receptor blockers (Avapro, Cozaar), calcium channel blockers (Norvasc), ACE inhibitors (Altace, Lotensin)
Birth control with high levels of progesterone (Depo-Provera) or high estrogen (Ortho Evra)	For women with severe diabetes, high levels of estrogen in certain meds may raise blood sugar; progesterone can increase insulin resistance.	Low-dose pills, such as Mircette and Ortho Tri-Cyclen Lo, or a hormone-free option like the ParaGard IUD

If you want...	Log on to...	Cost	The Basics
Expert advice at your fingertips	Mayo Clinic Health Manager (www. healthmanager. mayoclinic.com)	Free	Powered by Microsoft HealthVault, this service provides tips from some of the nation's top doctors. If you enter certain conditions—such as diabetes, asthma, or high blood pressure—the site offers up-to-date treatment information.
To share health records with your family	Google Health (www.google.com/ health)	Free	Anyone can sign up, but if you have a Google account, you're already halfway there. It's easy to store health records and share them with others you select, such as your spouse. Print a wallet-size version of your health profile to keep on hand for emergencies.
Reminders to keep your health on track	MyMediConnect (www.mymedi connect.net)	Free	This system has extra perks: It can send recorded reminders to take certain medications (you can have messages sent directly to any phone number), and members get news updates from the *Harvard Health Letter*.

Save Your Drug Money

Buying prescription meds in bulk can keep your wallet healthy, according to a recent University of Chicago study. Researchers found that people spent, on average, $15.10 per month when they bought a 3-month supply of drugs, compared with $20.44 for a single month's supply. That's a savings of nearly 30 percent.

"As long as your insurance allows it, there's little reason not to get a bigger supply of medicine that you are taking long-term," says study author G. Caleb Alexander, MD, an assistant professor in the department of medicine.

OPEN PILL BOTTLES WITH EASE

If you're routinely frustrated by impenetrable pill packaging—such as the hard plastic surrounding many over-the-counter medications—drop the steak knife and pick up the Popper. This handheld contraption quickly and safely frees individually packaged tablets. The Popper requires minimal dexterity and strength, and it works effectively on even the smallest blister packs or foil drug encasements.

The Popper costs $25 at www.freethepill.com, where there's also a 30-second how-to-use video.

■ GET FASTER, EASIER, SAFER CARE

Online personal health records (PHR) were once offered primarily by employers and insurers. But now they are available from private companies, some for free. A PHR won't just organize your life; it might also help save it during an emergency or make switching doctors easier, according to *Prevention* advisor David L. Katz, MD, director of the Yale-Griffin Prevention Research Center in Derby, Connecticut.

Don't worry about privacy: Most sites securely encrypt your data, making it inaccessible to outsiders and advertisers.

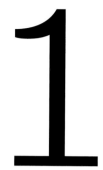

FIGHT
Diabetes Right

Only you have the power to control your diabetes.

Here's why—and how.

Diabetes is on the rise in the United States, and it shows no sign of slowing down. The latest data from the Centers for Disease Control and Prevention suggest that as many as 24 million Americans—a staggering number that's around the population of the Lone Star State—have some form of diabetes, mostly type 2 diabetes. According to the same study, another 57 million Americans have prediabetes, which raises the risk of developing the full-blown disease. Wherever you are on the diabetes spectrum, you've got plenty of company.

The good news is that type 2 diabetes is largely a lifestyle disease. It's true that genetics plays a role, as do environmental factors. But lifestyle is what tips the scale in one direction or the other—toward health or toward disease. For example, overweight, obesity, and excess belly fat are all powerful predictors of type 2. Those lifestyle factors are largely within your control. You can prevent prediabetes—or even stop it before it advances to full-blown diabetes. If you already have type 2, losing weight might help you avoid or delay the use of diabetes medications, and it might also reduce your risk of complications.

Both prediabetes and type 2 diabetes involve insulin resistance, which means that the muscle, liver, and fat cells don't properly use insulin, the hormone that helps usher glucose (sugar) from the bloodstream into cells. Once there, glucose is converted to energy. When cells are insulin resistant, glucose builds up in the bloodstream. Meanwhile, cells aren't getting the fuel they need to carry out their basic functions.

In prediabetes, the pancreas secretes more insulin to try to sweep the extra glucose out of the bloodstream. Eventually, though, it just can't keep up. This marks the onset of type 2, which doctors diagnose at or above a fasting blood glucose level of 126 mg/dL. Prediabetes refers to higher-than-normal fasting blood glucose, in the range of 100 to 125 mg/dL. Though it isn't the full-blown disease, it can lay the groundwork for complications later on. This is all the more reason to take action now, before it has a chance to do harm.

Blood Sugar Control

Do you know your blood sugar level? Most Americans have no idea. Yet many experts believe that knowing your blood sugar level is as important as knowing your telephone number and your e-mail address!

The American Diabetes Association recommends that people begin diabetes screening at age 45—even earlier if you're at risk. But thanks to the rise in obesity and the drop in physical activity in the United States, "earlier" now applies to most of us.

You should get checked right away if

you're carrying a few extra pounds and have even one of the diabetes risk factors: an inactive lifestyle; a family history of diabetes; a personal history of high blood pressure, low HDL, high triglycerides, diabetes during pregnancy, and/or polycystic ovary syndrome; and African American, Asian American, Latino, Native American, or Pacific Islander ancestry.

Some experts recommend testing even earlier. The American College of Endocrinology, an association of physicians who specialize in hormonal disorders including diabetes, recommends starting in your thirties. If type 2 diabetes runs strongly in your family, then testing beginning in your twenties makes sense.

Getting that first blood sugar measurement is critical. If you learn that you have diabetes, maintaining healthy blood sugar levels is the way to lower your risk for serious and even life-threatening complications such as heart attack, stroke, high blood pressure, kidney failure, nerve damage, vision loss, and amputation. If you're at risk for diabetes, a blood sugar check is the only way to find out whether or not you have prediabetes or have already developed full-blown type 2 diabetes—or if your blood sugar is still at a healthy level.

Here's why that blood sugar check is so important: Diabetes often has no symptoms. You might not feel any different as your blood sugar levels rise. This is the reason nearly six million people in the United States have type 2 diabetes

but don't know it—and why tens of millions more have prediabetes, the step before full-blown diabetes, yet are unaware of it.

Watching your diet and controlling your weight will shave points off your blood sugar reading, both directly and indirectly—in the latter case, by helping to trim your waistline. As your blood sugar stabilizes at a healthy level, you'll notice other changes, too. You'll feel more energized, you'll concentrate better, your mood will be brighter, and your food cravings should all but disappear.

Maybe these benefits will provide a little motivation for you to be extra vigilant about your blood sugar. We can't overstate the importance of maintaining

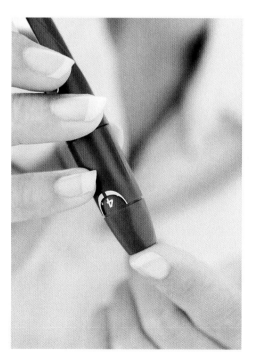

LEARN YOUR —————
DIABETES ABCS

Here's how people with diabetes say their ABCs.

A is for the A1C test, which tells you how effective your blood sugar control has been over the past 3 months. For most people with diabetes, the A1C goal is less than 7 percent.

B is for blood pressure. Shoot for 130/80 mm Hg or lower.

C is for cholesterol. Aim for a "bad" LDL cholesterol reading of less than 100 mg/dL.

good blood sugar control, especially in terms of the long-term health implications of type 2 diabetes. There's excellent research to illustrate how your risk of diabetes complications can rise and fall along with your blood sugar level.

A number of high-profile studies have explored the effects of what's known as intensive therapy, in which blood sugar is kept as close to normal as possible through a combination of oral medication, injected insulin, healthy lifestyle changes, and frequent interaction with health care providers.

One landmark study, known as the Diabetes Control and Complications Trial (DCCT), found that intensive blood sugar control reduced the risk of kidney disease by 34 percent, of diabetic neuropathy (nerve disease) by 60 percent, and of diabetic retinopathy (eye disease) by a phenomenal 76 percent.

A second study, called the ADVANCE trial—a large-scale, multicountry study conducted by Australian researchers—found that participants with type 2 diabetes who practiced intensive blood sugar control lowered their risk of kidney disease by a respectable 21 percent.

A third study, the Veterans Affairs Diabetes Trial (VADT), involved 1,791 US veterans (mostly male; average age, 60) who were assigned to standard- or intensive-treatment groups, both with a goal A1C reading of less than 7 percent (see page 13 for more about A1C levels). The participants started the trial with an average A1C of 9.5 percent; within 6 months, the average dropped to 6.9 percent among those receiving intensive treatment, compared with 8.4 percent among those getting standard treatment. Both groups were able to maintain their A1C levels for the duration of the trial.

These study outcomes have prompted diabetes experts to rethink the conventional wisdom on the use of intensive therapy as a means of preventing heart problems in those with diabetes. The consensus is that ultra-aggressive treatment to lower blood sugar simply isn't necessary, and neither are changes in the treatment guidelines.

What does all this research mean for you? First and foremost, it's vital to maintain good blood sugar control, regardless of whether you have diabetes or prediabetes. Losing weight, eating healthfully, and exercising regularly will make a huge difference in how effectively you keep your blood sugar in check.

Second, medication isn't the only answer to blood sugar trouble in most cases. This last caveat is important, because we know that some people simply can't stabilize their blood sugar without meds. But watching your diet and weight might help you reduce the amount of medication you require on a daily basis. (Don't ever change your dosage or stop taking medication without consulting your doctor.) And if you aren't using diabetes drugs yet, you might be able to avoid them altogether, especially if you're prediabetic.

Third, don't let your blood sugar control you. Too often, people with diabetes or prediabetes are so vigilant about managing their blood sugar that it becomes an all-consuming task. It is important, but it shouldn't drain the enjoyment and pleasure out of life.

Here are the ways you and your doctor will check your blood sugar levels.

FASTING BLOOD SUGAR TEST

Long the gold standard for diagnosing diabetes and prediabetes, the fasting blood sugar test (also called a fasting plasma glucose test) is quick and only a little inconvenient. You can't eat for 8 to 12 hours before your blood is drawn.

Schedule your test for the morning for best results. Studies show that morning tests are twice as likely as afternoon tests to catch blood sugar problems. The reason is that waiting until afternoon usu-ally means fasting for more than 12 hours, and blood sugar levels often drop precipitously after people have gone 14 or more hours without food. So while a morning test might turn up prediabetes or even full-blown diabetes, the evidence could disappear by midafternoon because your body has used up the excess blood sugar for energy.

What the Results Mean

Healthy: 70 to 99 mg/dL
Prediabetes: 100 to 125 mg/dL
Diabetes: 126 mg/dL and above

When to Retest

Doctors usually test twice to confirm a diagnosis of diabetes. We recommend retesting at least once a year if you're at risk of diabetes.

ORAL GLUCOSE TOLERANCE TEST

This check, which tests your body's response to blood sugar immediately after a meal, takes longer than the fasting blood glucose test—more than 2 hours from start to finish. It can be a more sensitive way to detect prediabetes and to assess whether prediabetes is progressing toward diabetes. For these reasons, the American Diabetes Association says it can be used in place of a fasting blood sugar test. Some doctors use this test in addition to a fasting check to look for high blood sugar levels after a meal that a fasting test might miss.

For this test, after an overnight fast (8 to 12 hours or so), you report to the doctor's office or lab. A blood sample is taken (to check fasting blood sugar), then you drink a very sweet beverage (sort of like a flat cola or orange soda, but thicker) containing 75 milligrams of glucose. Your blood is drawn after 1 hour and again after 2 hours. Bring something to read because you'll be sitting in a waiting room between blood draws. Blood glucose (blood sugar) levels of both blood samples will be checked.

What the Results Mean
Normal: Less than 140 mg/dL
Prediabetes: From 140 to 200 mg/dL
Diabetes: Over 200 mg/dL

When to Retest
Doctors usually test twice to confirm a diagnosis of diabetes. We recommend rechecking once a year if you're at risk for diabetes.

DAILY GLUCOSE MONITORING
If you have prediabetes or diabetes, you're likely monitoring your glucose very carefully. To use your glucose monitor—also called a blood sugar meter or glucometer—just prick your finger for a blood sample, and you get nearly instant feedback about your blood sugar level. These checks are a cornerstone of stellar blood sugar control because they give you immediate, real-time information about how the sandwich you just ate for lunch, the medication you took 2 hours ago, the walk you just enjoyed, or even relaxation

Make a List
Create a list of your support team's telephone numbers and e-mail addresses—including your primary care physician, nutritionist, dentist, podiatrist, and pharmacist. This way, you'll be able to reach them quickly and easily if you have a question. Place one copy of your list in your wallet and another by your home telephone. If you don't have a support team, talk to your doctor about assembling one.

exercises affect your blood sugar. This information empowers you to make smart decisions that help keep your blood sugar within a healthy range.

Glucose checks are good for revealing your blood sugar level at one moment in time. Daily tests are like snapshots and are extremely useful for finding out how high your blood sugar is at key times of the day: first thing in the morning before you eat, before a meal, and before and after exercise. They also let you see how well your body handles the natural rise in blood sugar after you eat. These checks give you up-to-the-minute info on how your meal choices and portions, physical activity, stress levels, and medications affect your blood sugar. Regular checks are vital if you take insulin or other diabetes medications, have low blood sugar episodes without warning signs, or have a difficult time controlling your diabetes.

What the Results Mean

Ideal on a fasting test or before a meal: 90 to 130 mg/dL

Ideal 2 hours after the beginning of a meal: Less than 180 mg/dL

When to Retest

Retest as recommended by your doctor. Some people test many times each day; others with well-controlled blood sugar test just a few times a week.

A1C LEVELS

An A1C check, which is usually done in your doctor's office, tells you what your blood sugar "batting average" is. It's a sign of your overall blood sugar level for the past 2 to 3 months and clues you in on how well your blood sugar was controlled around the clock, every day. High levels over many years increase your risk of diabetes complications. On the other hand, in-control levels reduce it.

The A1C tells you how much blood sugar has attached itself to hemoglobin molecules in your red blood cells. The more sugarcoated hemoglobin you have, the higher your A1C percentage is. Home tests are available and can be convenient, but be sure to share the results every time with your doctor and your diabetes care team so that changes can be made in your diabetes management plan if needed.

These checks are good for seeing whether your diabetes management plan is really working. They're not helpful for judging how your blood sugar responds to specific meals, foods, exercise sessions, or a single dose of medication, however.

What the Results Mean

Ideal: Below 6.5 percent if recommended by your doctor

Healthy: Below 7 percent

High: Above 7 percent for most people with diabetes

When to Retest

Each person's goal may be different, so be sure to discuss retesting with your doctor. Generally, doctors test two to four times a year.

Know Your Other Numbers, Too

Managing diabetes means maintaining healthy blood sugar levels, but it also means taking your cholesterol, triglyceride, and blood pressure levels seriously.

One of the most stunning facts about diabetes, prediabetes, and metabolic syndrome (a step before prediabetes) is how these conditions also raise your risk of heart attacks and strokes. That's why the American Diabetes Association says it's vital for people with diabetes to know their blood pressure, cholesterol, and triglyceride levels—and keep them in a healthy range. Knowing these numbers is equally important if you're at risk of diabetes because it can even tip you off to early body-chemistry changes that may lead to diabetes.

If you know your blood sugar, cholesterol, and blood pressure levels, you'll feel more in control. You and your doctor have the information you need to take the next steps. You don't have to worry any longer. You know where you stand, and you're ready to take action.

Your doctor or health care practitioner will most likely check these numbers and give you a fasting blood sugar test. If not, ask her to do so. And there's emerging evidence that for people with diabetes, these numbers are not just important

MYSTERIOUS METABOLIC SYNDROME

Metabolic syndrome is a cluster of symptoms that can often precede diabetes. It might look like a bunch of little, unrelated health problems, but it's a sign that you have insulin resistance—the driving force behind type 2 diabetes. Don't ignore it. Even if your blood sugar is still in the normal range, having metabolic syndrome boosts your risk of eventually developing diabetes 5 times higher, and your risk for cardiovascular disease 1.6 to 2 times higher, than it is for people who do not have metabolic syndrome.

The more of this health condition's signature traits you have, the higher your risk. Compared with three traits, having five traits raised diabetes risk twice as high—to 10 times higher than normal—in one British study.

You have metabolic syndrome if you have any three of the following:

- A waist measurement of 40 inches or more for men and 35 inches or more for women
- Triglyceride levels of 150 milligrams per deciliter (mg/dL) or above, or if you are taking medication for elevated triglyceride levels
- An HDL, or "good," cholesterol level below 40 mg/dL for men and below 50 mg/dL for women, or if you are taking medication for low HDL levels
- A blood pressure level of 130/85 or above, or if you are taking medication for elevated blood pressure levels
- Fasting blood sugar levels of 100 mg/dL or above, or if you are taking medication for elevated blood glucose levels

If you have metabolic syndrome, many experts say that lifestyle changes, such as watching your diet and your weight, are usually the first choice for taming the condition, but be sure to get your doctor involved. She can advise you about the best ways to raise your HDLs, control your blood pressure, and lower your triglycerides. Ask how often you should have these risk factors rechecked to see if they're returning to normal.

indicators of the health of your cardiovascular system. They may also indicate your risk for nerve damage, which is a complication experienced by three out of five people with diabetes. If you do not have diabetes, they also help determine whether you have metabolic syndrome, a condition that begins raising your risk for diabetes even if your blood sugar levels look normal.

If any of these numbers are high, your doctor might suggest starting with healthy lifestyle changes—weight loss, exercise, healthful eating—and may or may not prescribe medication to help you reach healthy targets. You might be rechecked in 3 to 6 months. How often should you be retested after that? Your doctor will probably check your blood pressure at every visit—and at the very least, once a year. Experts recommend that people who do not have diabetes get their cholesterol and triglycerides checked at least once every 5 years, and more often if those levels have ever been high. If you have diabetes, they should be checked annually.

BLOOD PRESSURE

Hypertension, or high blood pressure, damages arteries and raises your risk of heart attack and stroke. It also contributes to kidney failure if you have diabetes. The top number, called systolic pressure, measures pressure during a heartbeat. The bottom measures diastolic pressure, which is the force of blood through your arteries between beats. All measurements are in millimeters of mercury.

What the Results Mean

Low blood pressure: Below 90/60 mm Hg
Healthy: 119/79 mm Hg to 90/60 mm Hg (115/75 mm Hg is ideal)
Prehypertension: 120/80 mm Hg to 139/89 mm Hg
Hypertension: 140/90 mm Hg and above

When to Retest

At least once a year; recheck after 3 to 6 months if you're trying to lower your blood pressure with healthy lifestyle changes.

LDL CHOLESTEROL

"Bad" LDL cholesterol packs heart-threatening plaque into artery walls, raising your odds of a heart attack or stroke. It also contributes to circulation problems, which are already a concern for people with diabetes, especially in the legs and feet.

What the Results Mean

Ideal: Less than 100 mg/dL
Healthy: 100 to 129 mg/dL
Borderline high: 130 to 159 mg/dL
High: 160 to 189 mg/dL
Very high: 190 mg/dL and above

When to Retest

Repeat every 5 years if normal—after 3 to 6 months if you're using healthy lifestyle changes to lower high LDL.

HDL CHOLESTEROL

This "good" cholesterol protects against heart attack and stroke by ferrying "bad" LDL to the liver for elimination. When HDL is low, your body can't eliminate LDL effectively. This raises your risk of heart attacks and strokes.

What the Results Mean

Low: Below 50 mg/dL for women, below 40 mg/dL for men

Healthy: 50 mg/dL and over for women, 40 mg/dL and over for men

Ideal: 60 mg/dL and above

When to Retest

Repeat every 5 years if normal—after 3 to 6 months if you're using healthy lifestyle changes to improve HDL levels.

TRIGLYCERIDES

Normally, this blood fat carries extra fat from the food you eat to fat cells for storage. But if you eat too much fat or too many calories, your liver converts the excess into an overabundance of triglycerides—then uses them as raw material for making small, dense LDLs, an extralethal type of LDL that accelerates growth of plaque in artery walls. At high levels, these blood fats raise heart attack and stroke risk.

If you have diabetes, high triglycerides are troublesome for another reason. They seem to go hand in hand with extra risk of nerve damage, University of Michigan researchers report in a new study. In fact, the researchers recommend that people with diabetes be as careful with their triglycerides as they are with their blood sugar.

What the Results Mean

Normal: Less than 150 mg/dL

Borderline high: 150–199 mg/dL

High: 200–499 mg/dL

Very high: 500 mg/dL and above

When to Retest

Repeat every 5 years if normal—after 3 to 6 months if you're using healthy lifestyle changes to lower high levels of triglycerides.

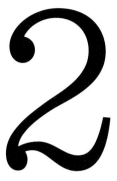

Choose Your BEST CURE

Most drugs and therapies fail in half of all patients. **Here's how to figure out what will work for you,** taking into account diabetes and its complications.

You hear the pitch in drug ads all the time: "Ask your doctor if this medication is right for you." Trouble is, in many cases the only way your doctor can answer the question is by having you try the drug. And as the latest research reveals, what's "right" for the smiling folks in a TV commercial may be just plain wrong for you.

One reason: Each of us responds uniquely to any given medication. "Your liver and kidney function, overall health, treatment for other conditions, and genetics all play a role in how a drug affects you," says Martha Gerrity, MD, PhD, clinical evidence specialist at the Center for Evidence-Based Policy at Oregon Health & Science University (OHSU) in Portland.

Another reason: The chances of your having a good response are simply not in your favor. "To market a medication, all you have to do is prove that it's better, on average, than a sugar pill," says John Mark Gibson, director of the OHSU center. A drug that works 20 percent of the time, for instance, might be considered effective—even though it does nothing for 80 percent of patients.

Those odds could improve soon, thanks to a national push to comb through studies and scientific reviews to determine who gets better most often on which drugs. Called comparative effectiveness research, the initiative aims to produce a reliable set of guidelines that will enable you and your doctor to choose treatments based on solid evidence, not guesswork. The Obama administration has made comparative effectiveness research a pri-

ority, funneling more than $1 billion—"a huge increase," says Gibson—into the program as part of the government's stimulus package.

Already, 28 research centers funded by the government's Agency for Healthcare Research and Quality (AHRQ) have produced a wealth of findings on treatments for many common, chronic conditions. If you suffer from one of them, first start with lifestyle changes such as exercise and a modified diet. Then, when you're ready to try drug treatment, talk to your doctor about the steps outlined here—all supported by powerful new research.

Type 2 Diabetes

Diet, exercise, and weight control are among the most potent tools for bringing down high blood sugar. A 10-pound weight loss—even in someone who is obese—can help patients with diabetes as much as adding another medication can, according to Dr. Gerrity. A variety of drugs also effectively control blood sugar.

First, try metformin (Glucophage), which decreases the amount of glucose absorbed from food and made by the liver. Metformin is older and cheaper than many other drugs, but it matches or outperforms the newer thiazolidinediones (Actos, Avandia), according to a new review.

If that doesn't work, combine metformin with a second drug, such as a sulfonylurea, which increases the body's insulin production.

"Because metformin and sulfonylureas work in different ways, the drugs lower blood sugar together better than either drug would by itself," says Dr. Gerrity.

TAILOR YOUR TREATMENT

If you're overweight, stick to metformin; it won't make you gain weight.

If you have high cholesterol, avoid Avandia and Actos, which can raise bad LDL cholesterol and worsen congestive heart failure, according to AHRQ reports. Opt for metformin, which can lower LDL.

If you have a sensitive stomach, take a smaller dose of metformin, which is more likely than other diabetes pills to cause diarrhea and stomach cramps. If the lower dose proves less effective, combine metformin with a different drug to keep blood sugar under control.

GO NATURAL

"Eat high-fiber, unprocessed foods, especially legumes," advises Kevin A. Barrows, MD, director of clinical programs at the Osher Center for Integrative Medicine at the University of California, San Francisco. Some reports suggest that you can also lower blood sugar by taking the botanicals *Gymnema sylvestre* and bitter melon, but don't combine them with prescription meds.

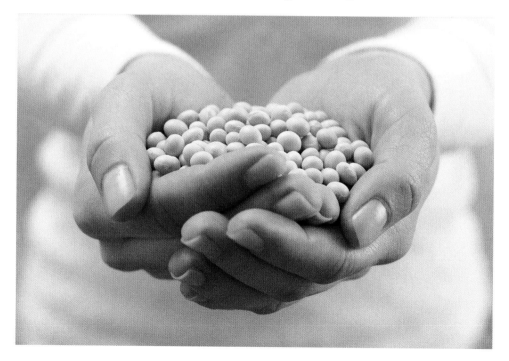

High Blood Pressure

According to the American Diabetes Association, as many as two out of three adults with diabetes have blood pressure, which can increase your risk of heart attack, stroke, eye problems, and kidney problems.

If you're overweight, you can lower your blood pressure by losing just 5 pounds. And each healthy strategy for dropping those pounds—exercising; consuming less saturated fat; eating more fruits, vegetables, and whole grains—can help tame hypertension. But you may still need med-

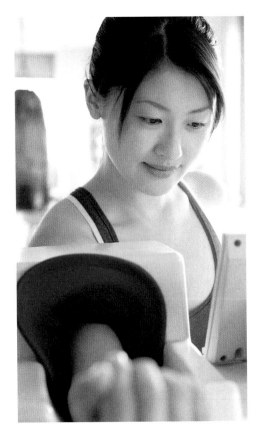

ical treatment, depending in part on how high your blood pressure is.

First, try a diuretic, which takes pressure off blood vessels by making the body eliminate water and sodium. "Many people with hypertension who take a diuretic alone are able to bring blood pressure down to a target of 130/90 or, ideally, 120/80, with relatively few side effects," says Dr. Gerrity.

If that doesn't work, take a two-pronged approach by adding a beta-blocker, ACE inhibitor, or angiotensin II receptor blocker, all of which work in a manner different from that of your diuretic.

TAILOR YOUR TREATMENT

If you have kidney problems, make your second drug an ACE inhibitor, which protects the kidneys.

If you're African American, consider starting with a combination treatment that includes a diuretic. African Americans generally don't respond as well to treatment with just one drug.

If your blood pressure is really high—systolic pressure 160 or higher, or diastolic pressure 100 or higher—start right away with combo treatment to bring it down quickly.

If you have ischemic heart disease, which can cause your pulse to be irregular or rapid, instead of a diuretic, start with a beta-blocker, which can help lower your heart rate.

If you're pregnant, avoid ACE inhibitors and angiotensin II receptor blockers; they can cause birth defects. Better choices: beta-blockers and vasodilators that relax blood vessels.

GO NATURAL

Omega-3 fatty acids lower blood pressure, but only in high doses (above 3 grams a day) that may increase your risk of bleeding, so take them only under a doctor's supervision.

Coenzyme Q10 may also cause small drops in blood pressure and may lower blood sugar levels in some people, so be cautious if you're taking diabetes medication.

Depression

People who have diabetes are at a greater risk of depression. Plus, poor diabetes control can cause symptoms that mimic depression.

Exercise can brighten your blues by reducing stress, releasing muscle tension, building self-esteem, helping you sleep, and boosting levels of feel-good brain chemicals. But you may need treatment to help get you going if you're feeling listless. Six out of 10 people feel better on the first antidepressant they try; the rest need to try other drugs, according to the AHRQ. Ask your doctor about the cytochrome P450 genotyping test, which is a genetic analysis that can help you predict which drugs will work best for you and whether you're more likely to experience side effects.

First, try a selective serotonin reuptake inhibitor (SSRI), such as fluoxetine (Prozac, Sarafem), paroxetine (Paxil), or sertraline (Zoloft). Most people feel that these drugs help, and research has found that they have fewer side effects than other antidepressants.

If that doesn't work, tricyclic antidepressants work as well as SSRIs do, although side effects are usually more numerous and severe.

TAILOR YOUR TREATMENT

If you're overweight, avoid paroxetine and mirtazapine (Remeron), which are more likely to cause weight gain than drugs like fluoxetine and sertraline, according to a government report. Consider bupropion (Wellbutrin), which tends to shave off 2 or 3 pounds.

If you have sexual problems, bupropion is less likely to cause loss of desire or trouble reaching orgasm than fluoxetine, sertraline, and especially paroxetine.

If you also take drugs for diabetes or high blood pressure, watch glucose and blood pressure levels more closely. Both sulfonylureas and beta-blockers use the same chemical pathways in the liver as antidepressants, so starting an SSRI may increase or decrease the potency of these medications, Dr. Gerrity advises.

GO NATURAL

Supplements of SAM-e, which is a naturally occurring building block of brain chemicals (such as serotonin) that help stabilize mood, were found to significantly boost patients' spirits in an AHRQ review of 28 studies.

Joint Pain

Wondering if there's a connection between joint pain and diabetes? Certainly: Many people with diabetes are overweight, and being overweight increases joint pain.

Staying active should be a lifelong strategy: Walking and other moderate exercise can reduce pain, keep you flexible, and strengthen muscles supporting your joints. However, many people who suffer from joint pain find that they need more help.

First, try methotrexate for rheumatoid arthritis. Called a DMARD (disease-modifying antirheumatic drug), it suppresses the immune system attacks that characterize the disease, tamping down the inflammation that causes joint damage and pain. It also comes in a pill that can be as effective as similar drugs delivered in shots or IV treatments, according to a new government guide. If your pain is caused by osteoarthritis, start with acetaminophen (Tylenol), the over-the-counter (OTC) painkiller that's least likely to cause side effects.

If that doesn't work, a combo of methotrexate and a DMARD injection usually works better than methotrexate pills alone for people with more aggressive and drug-resistant rheumatoid arthritis. Don't double up with another oral DMARD, because research shows that pills generally aren't more effective together than they are alone. For osteoarthritis, try naproxen (Aleve, Naprosyn), which is a nonsteroidal anti-inflammatory drug (NSAID) that doesn't increase your chances of a heart attack the way celecoxib (Celebrex) and diclofenac (Voltaren) do.

TAILOR YOUR TREATMENT

If you're at risk of heart disease, avoid ibuprofen (Advil, Motrin): It poses cardiovascular risks for more people than other anti-inflammatories do, reports the American College of Rheumatology.

If you're over age 45, try to use anti-inflammatories sparingly. At least three times as many people in this age group experience serious stomach bleeding, compared with younger adults taking these drugs.

If you're premenopausal, use two forms of birth control (such as the Pill plus a condom) while taking methotrexate, which can cause serious birth defects.

GO NATURAL

Try fish oil supplements containing omega-3 fatty acids for rheumatoid arthritis. "Fish oil appears to be a potent anti-inflammatory," says Dr. Barrows. He recommends 3 grams of omega-3s daily, possibly increasing to 6 grams if needed, so check the appropriate amount with your doctor. For osteoarthritis, glucosamine hydrochloride with chondroitin sulfate may ease moderate to severe pain with few possible side effects, according to the AHRQ.

"Although some recent research concluded chondroitin doesn't help, far more studies have shown that it does," says Dr. Barrows.

Poor Sleep

Insomnia is one of the most common complaints in America, and it also has a link to diabetes: Sleep deprivation can make diabetes worse, and diabetes symptoms can make it harder to sleep.

Nondrug solutions can work as well as or better than medication for insomnia, although they may take 1 to 3 weeks to become effective. One recent review of 37 studies found that mental techniques such as trying to stay awake instead of trying to fall asleep—a reverse psychology technique known as paradoxical intention—consistently helped people with insomnia nod off. But resistant sleep problems often need to be addressed with drugs.

First, try zolpidem (Ambien). "It's effective in 75 to 80 percent of people who try it and is generally safe," says James K. Walsh, PhD, executive director and senior scientist at the Sleep Medicine and Research Center at St. Luke's Hospital in Chesterfield, Missouri.

If that doesn't work, try a longer-acting sleep medication, such as eszopiclone (Lunesta) or Ambien CR, both of which are active in the body for approximately 8 hours.

TAILOR YOUR TREATMENT

If you have trouble falling asleep, you'll nod off faster after taking zaleplon (Sonata) than you will if you take Ambien, according to a review by the Oregon Evidence-Based Practice Center at OHSU.

If you awake during the night, Ambien, Lunesta, and other sleep medications tend to provide longer periods of sleep than Sonata and keep people asleep once slumber overtakes them.

GO NATURAL

"Cognitive behavioral therapy [CBT] can work as well as drugs, and its effects last up to 6 months after you stop treatment," says Dr. Walsh.

In CBT, you redirect your mind away from anxiety-producing thoughts and start spending less time in bed, not more. That makes you more tired the next time you hit the sack, so sleep comes easier. "Once you're sleeping better, you can start sleeping longer," Dr. Walsh explains.

Go to www.nacbt.org to search for a therapist.

Migraines

Although there might not be a direct connection between diabetes and migraines, people with diabetes get migraines just as often as the rest of us do.

Keeping a headache diary is one of the best ways to identify your triggers and possibly prevent future attacks. It also helps your doctor find a prevention and treatment plan that works for you. Record possible food triggers, emotional stress, alcohol consumption, medication, hormonal changes, and sleep patterns.

Still, the throbbing onslaught of headache pain can be difficult to predict, so a variety of drugs have been developed specifically to treat migraines—and some designed for other conditions might help as well.

First, try an OTC or prescription NSAID such as ibuprofen, or a combo drug such as Excedrin Migraine, which contains acetaminophen, aspirin, and caffeine. These drugs will often relieve mild to moderate migraine pain but may not help a severe attack, according to guidelines from the American Academy of Neurology.

"Take an NSAID as soon as you feel a migraine coming on," says Dr. Gerrity. "It's more effective at the beginning of the headache."

If that doesn't work, try a triptan, such as sumatriptan (Imitrex) or rizatriptan (Maxalt), which can relieve pain, nausea, and sensitivity to light but has relatively few side effects. Research shows that sumatriptan works especially well when taken with naproxen (an NSAID). And a review from the Oregon Evidence-Based Practice Center found rizatriptan especially effective at providing 2-hour relief, compared with sumatriptan and naratriptan (Amerge).

TAILOR YOUR TREATMENT

If you're treating high blood pressure, consider using beta-blockers, which can make migraines milder and less frequent. If that doesn't help, try a calcium channel blocker, such as verapamil (Calan, Isoptin), which is another type of high blood pressure medication that might also relieve migraines.

If migraines strike more than twice a month, try a medication shown to prevent migraines, such as a tricyclic antidepressant or an antiseizure drug like topiramate (Topamax).

GO NATURAL

There's good evidence that butterbur is an effective supplement in treating migraine pain. And magnesium supplements might make migraines less frequent by correcting deficiencies that seem to be more common in migraine sufferers.

"Feverfew and riboflavin may also help," says Dr. Barrows. Combination products such as MigreLief put magnesium, feverfew, and riboflavin in a single pill.

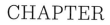

CHAPTER

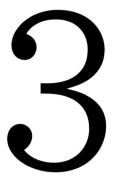

3

Beware of Shadow

DISEASES

Experts aren't sure why some illnesses travel in pairs, such as diabetes and high blood pressure. **Knowing your risk will help you stay safe.**

For years, doctors have observed that patients with one illness may be stricken by another condition that's seemingly unrelated and sometimes more serious, known as a shadow disease. One of the most well-known connections is that between migraines and heart attack or stroke. Now researchers are uncovering even more linked ailments and zeroing in on why they appear to travel in pairs.

Studies show that these couplings occur for different reasons. In some cases, one disease creates damage that causes the second illness. In others, troublesome genes or poor health behaviors, such as smoking and lack of exercise, trigger one problem, then the other. Being alert to the dangerous connections described below can help you avoid the shadow disease or get early diagnosis and treatment, leading to a better outcome.

High Blood Pressure's Shadow: Diabetes

Doctors have long wondered how high blood pressure and diabetes are related because the two often appear together, especially in obese patients. Now, after following 38,000 midlife women for 10 years, researchers at Brigham and Women's Hospital and Harvard Medical School report that constantly elevated blood pressure, or hypertension, doubles your risk of developing diabetes, regardless of your body mass index. More surprising, the risk of diabetes goes up if your blood pressure increases over time— even if it stays under the hypertension threshold.

The two problems may have a common cause, according to study author David Conen, MD, a research fellow at Brigham and Women's Hospital. Potential culprits include high levels of inflammation in the body, he says, or a malfunction in the blood vessels' inner lining, allowing blood cells to leak into surrounding tissue and damage it.

PROTECT YOURSELF

If you have mild hypertension or are at risk of this problem, get tested for diabetes. You can help prevent the onset of diabetes with lifestyle changes: Increase your physical activity, lose excess weight, limit salt, and stub out those cigarettes for good, suggests Dr. Conen.

Metabolic Syndrome's Shadow: Kidney Stones

Metabolic syndrome is a serious health condition associated with diabetes, coronary heart attacks, and even early death. You have it if you've got at least three of these five traits: excess abdominal fat, high blood triglycerides, low HDL (the good cholesterol), high blood pressure, and impaired glucose tolerance.

Now a new study reveals that metabolic syndrome could also be behind the rising rate of kidney stones. Your odds of developing them go up by 54 percent if you have two of the above traits. With three symptoms, your risk hits 70 percent, according to the research.

PROTECT YOURSELF

Obesity is a key player in both metabolic syndrome and kidney stones, perhaps because overweight people are likely to consume excess protein and sodium, which may cause the painful crystals to develop, says study coauthor Bradford Lee West, MD. Trimming your waistline reduces one of the metabolic syndrome traits and might diminish your chances of getting kidney stones, he says.

Migraine's Shadow: Stroke or Heart Attack

If you regularly suffer from migraine pain (especially if you develop auras, which are visual or sensory phenomena that accompany the headache), your doctor has probably warned you about your susceptibility to heart attack or stroke. Now, thanks to findings announced in 2007, experts better understand which cardiac ailment is more likely to occur for any given migraine sufferer. This is especially important for people with diabetes, who are already at great risk of heart attack and stroke.

Frequency matters. If you have less than one migraine a month, you're 50 percent more likely than a nonsufferer to have a heart attack. If migraines strike at least weekly, you have three times the risk of stroke, compared with someone who doesn't have this problem, according to study coauthor Tobias Kurth, MD, an assistant professor at Harvard Medical School.

PROTECT YOURSELF

Unfortunately, existing research has not yet found that preventing migraines has the effect of lowering stroke or heart attack odds. However, by keeping your cardiovascular system as healthy as possible, you diminish your chance of a cardiac event, according to the National Stroke Association. To do this, control known hazards, such as high cholesterol and obesity, via diet and exercise. You should also quit smoking and limit alcohol intake. According to the American Heart Association, this means an average of one to two drinks per day for men and one drink per day for women. (A drink is one 12-ounce beer, 4 ounces of wine, 1.5 ounces of 80-proof spirits, or 1 ounce of 100-proof spirits.)

Endometriosis's Shadow: Melanoma

In 2007, a huge, 12-year French study confirmed that women who have endometriosis (in which tissue similar to the uterine lining grows outside the womb) are 62 percent more likely to suffer from melanoma. Researchers are unsure why endometriosis and the deadly skin cancer sometimes travel together, but one possibility is a genetic defect that triggers both conditions.

Why is this important to people with diabetes? Although it's rare, in people with diabetes melanomas can appear to be neuropathic foot ulcers and, therefore, not identified as early as they could be.

PROTECT YOURSELF

If you have endometriosis, ask your doctor to scan your skin for melanoma, advises Jeffrey P. Callen, MD, a professor of dermatology at the University of Louisville School of Medicine.

You can also do a self-check by comparing your moles with problem growths pictured at www.prevention.com/moles.

If anything suspicious turns up, be sure to have it biopsied. Don't panic, though. "When diagnosed very early, melanoma is nearly 100 percent curable," Dr. Callen says.

Psoriasis's Shadow: Heart Attack

The rough, itchy patches of psoriasis are more than uncomfortable and unsightly. According to a recent study, women with psoriasis are more likely to develop diabetes and also high blood pressure. To make matters even worse, those patches might increase odds of a heart attack, concluded a study that followed half a million people for 5 years. The risk of a cardiac emergency was related to the severity of the psoriasis, the researchers determined. Serious cases of the skin ailment could mean a more than doubled heart attack risk.

"The out-of-whack immune system that triggers the psoriasis may also cause inflammation that infiltrates the arteries of the heart," explains study author Joel M. Gelfand, MD, an assistant professor of dermatology at the University of Pennsylvania in Philadelphia.

PROTECT YOURSELF

Will controlling the skin disease diminish the inflammation that can cause a heart attack? The idea makes sense, but it must be confirmed with further research, says Dr. Gelfand. Consider talking with your doctor about new psoriasis medications, including alefacept (Amevive). They're made from living sources, much as vaccines are. They may work for you, even if past treatments have failed. In the meantime, Dr. Gelfand suggests, keep your heart healthy with diet and exercise.

Watch Out for the Great
DRUG SWITCHEROO

Your pharmacist might be changing your medication without your knowledge—and **what you don't know could worsen your diabetes and hurt you.** Here's how to stay safe.

When you hand a pharmacist a prescription, you expect to get the medication your doctor ordered. But because of a perfectly legal loophole in rules that govern how drugs are dispensed, you may not—and the consequences can be dire.

Just ask Amy Detrick of Grove City, Ohio. For months after the former social worker, 40, was diagnosed with epilepsy, her doctor fine-tuned the precise cocktail of meds that would keep her from having seizures—adding and subtracting drugs, calibrating doses, and carefully tracking how she responded. When her condition was finally under control, she filled a prescription for one of two drugs she took—Tegretol—and shortly afterward had a seizure while riding a bicycle. She fell off the bike, broke her leg, and had a hairline fracture in her left eye socket. While the doctors were treating her, they noticed that the blood level of her medication had declined. Her pharmacist, she learned, had exchanged her Tegretol for a generic that worked a little differently.

"Just imagine what could have happened had I been behind the wheel of a car," she says.

Detrick's story sounds like a medical mistake, but it wasn't. Instead, she experienced a potentially deadly consequence of a common practice called therapeutic substitution, wherein her pharmacist legally switched a drug prescribed by her doc, but without telling her or her physician. Usually, pharmacists replace a brand-name drug with a generic formula-

tion of the exact same medication. Therapeutic substitution is similar but with one crucial distinction: The new drug is in the same class as the old and treats the same condition, but it's not precisely the same medication.

To understand the nuance, think of statins. They constitute a single class of medication because they all lower cholesterol by reducing its production in the liver. But not every statin lowers cholesterol by the same amount or with the same balance of LDL to HDL. So if your doctor orders a brand name drug but your pharmacist switches it for the cheaper version of a different medication (but still a statin), you might not get the precise benefit your doctor had in mind—and may, in fact, suffer unexpected side effects.

In one way, at least, patients can benefit from substitution: smaller co-pays. But two-thirds of people who reported having meds switched in a National Consumers League (NCL) survey said they weren't consulted. Of those, 40 percent said the new drug was not as effective, and a third said it had more side effects.

"It's not okay for your insurance company or pharmacist to change your drugs without your knowledge," says NCL executive director Sally Greenberg.

Unfortunately, therapeutic substitution is likely here to stay—meaning you need to be on the lookout to make sure you're not harmed by the practice. Here are three common reasons you could end up with a less effective drug, and steps you can take to ensure that you get the medication to treat your condition properly.

Your Pharmacy Misreads the Law

After Tony Catizone of Chicago had a stroke while using a widely prescribed blood pressure medication, his doctor wrote a prescription for a new one, but a mail order pharmacy changed the prescription back to the old drug. His son, Carmen, caught the substitution and called the pharmacy.

"They told me that legally, they had to make the switch," says Carmen. Yet no state mandates therapeutic substitution, and even out-of-state mail-order houses must comply with the laws in your state. In Illinois, therapeutic substitution is allowed only in hospitals, where doctors control the process.

"The pharmacy was misinformed, evidently taking the insurer's list of covered drugs as the law," Carmen says. He knew this because he is executive director of the National Association of Boards of Pharmacy. "I told them I had a copy of the Illinois Practice Regulations and knew the law entitled my father to the right drug,"

he says. After transferring him from a customer service rep to a real pharmacist, the pharmacy corrected the switch.

GET THE RIGHT DRUG

- If your doctor believes her drug of choice should not be switched for another, ask her to write "medically necessary," "may not substitute," or "DAW"—for "dispense as written"—on the prescription. That obligates the pharmacist to check with you and your doctor before making any switches.

- If a pharmacy tells you the law requires a substitution, find out which ones your state allows and challenge the switch if

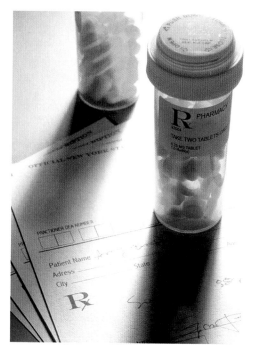

the pharmacy has overstepped its authority. To get the information you need, contact your state's board of pharmacy. Go to www.nabp.net and click on the Boards of Pharmacy button to bring up a contacts list for every state office.

- Pick a pharmacy you like and stick with it. "That way, your pharmacy will have a long record of your prescription history and know if a drug didn't work for you," says Carmen Catizone, whose father had stopped going to a neighborhood drugstore when his insurance company changed to mail-order prescriptions only.

- Ask your pharmacist to put a blanket statement in your records that you don't want any medications switched unless you and your doctor approve. "It's a way of getting your pharmacist's attention," says Catizone. "When pharmacists know more, they can do a better job of advocating for patients."

Your Insurance Company Refuses to Pay

Insurance plan formularies—the lists of drugs that insurers cover—are at the heart of most substitution battles.

"The insurance company will tell me that the drug I prescribed for a patient is not approved or is at the higher co-pay, so I need to submit documentation justifying why insurance should cover it instead of making a substitution," says Lori J. Heim, MD, president of the American Academy of Family Physicians. If a doctor persuades the insurance company that a particular drug is medically necessary, the insurer may cover it after all. But the haggling, follow-ups, and appeals can be time-consuming—and infuriating. One frustrated Ohio doctor sued Medco, a large pharmacy benefits management company, asking to be compensated for time wasted on prescription hassles—and won a small award. Court testimony in the case revealed that the company sent 57 times more prescription-related inquiries to physicians in 2007 than it did 10 years earlier.

Meanwhile, as doctors deal with an ocean of paperwork and bicker with insurers, patients suffer. "I've had patients who did not have control of their allergy symptoms—sneezing and feeling miserable—while I jumped through hoops showing that these other drugs didn't work for them," says Dr. Heim.

GET THE RIGHT DRUG

- Ask your doctor up front—before you fill your prescription—which generics, if any, are acceptable substitutions for the drug that she wants you to take. A switch at the pharmacy may be perfectly fine (and often cheaper for you). Write down the name of the prescribed medication and the approved subs on a piece of paper separate from the prescription slip, and then check the filled order against your list. If your pharmacist makes an unapproved switch, call your doctor right away so that he can begin documenting why insurance should cover the original drug or an appropriate alternative.

■ If your doctor doesn't fight a substitution, make sure he isn't just taking the path of least resistance or losing your prescription in the shuffle. "Busy doctors sign papers quickly, so it's easy for a substitution to sneak through," says Robert E. Reneker Jr., MD, urgent care physician at Spectrum Health, a hospital system in Grand Rapids, Michigan. Ask: Will the new drug work better? How will I know if it does or doesn't? Are side effects different from those associated with the original prescription? How will it interact

FOUR COMMON SWITCHES

Here are examples of cheaper therapeutic substitutions for brand-name drugs—identified by the National Consumers League—and how they may affect you.

If your doctor prescribes Lipitor, which is a cholesterol-lowering statin . . .

You might get simvastatin, the generic equivalent of Zocor, another statin.

The danger: Lipitor does a better job of lowering LDL (bad) cholesterol and triglycerides, but simvastatin is better at raising HDL (good) cholesterol, so one drug may not treat your main problem as well as the other.

If your doctor prescribes Lexapro, which is an antidepressant . . .

You might get citalopram, a generic version of the antidepressant Celexa.

The danger: You could experience more side effects with citalopram: Lexapro is more concentrated, so it's prescribed in smaller amounts.

If your doctor prescribes Diovan, which is an angiotensin receptor blocker for lowering blood pressure . . .

You might get lisinopril, the generic equivalent of Zestril, an ACE inhibitor for lowering blood pressure.

The danger: Patients on lisinopril sometimes develop a nagging cough.

If your doctor prescribes Nexium, which is a proton pump inhibitor for heartburn . . .

You might get omeprazole, the generic equivalent of Prilosec, an over-the-counter proton pump inhibitor.

The danger: Your body may respond better to one than the other; omeprazole may have more side effects.

with other medications or supplements I might be taking?

Your Pharmacy Cheats

You'd hope pharmacies are paragons of ethical behavior.

"But they're not always aboveboard," says Dr. Reneker. Sometimes, he says, pharmacies make drug switches because profit margins are higher on cheaper substitutes.

"Pharmacies are directly reimbursed by insurance companies and make more money from generics even though the sticker price for brand-name drugs is higher," says Dr. Reneker. "I've had pharmacies tell me a drug isn't on the formulary when I've already checked with the insurance company and know that it is.

The switch to a cheaper substitute is motivated purely by profit."

GET THE RIGHT DRUG

- Shop for prescriptions at stores that have slashed prices on generics—a move that lowers profit margins and reduces the temptation for pharmacists to make sneak switches. Giant retailers like Walmart and Target have led the way on price cuts, pressuring smaller pharmacies to match their discounts. "Drugs have become a way to attract people to stores so they'll spend money on other items," says Dr. Reneker.

- Call your insurance provider to confirm whether a drug is really covered if your pharmacist says it isn't.

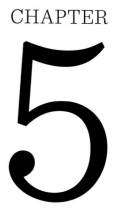

Don't Compound Your
PROBLEMS

Customized, compounded doses, types, and potencies of prescription medications aren't new, but they're unregulated by the FDA. Should you be worried? **Here's a *Prevention* special report on what you can do to protect your health.**

W hile going through menopause, Marcia Sticka developed miserable hot flashes and night sweats, dry skin, a short temper, and an uncharacteristic lack of energy. No more: Every day for the past 3 years, she's rubbed a low, precisely measured dose of the hormone testosterone onto her inner thighs, and she feels great.

"It really helped the hot flashes and night sweats, I'm not cranky all the time, and I wake up raring to go," says Sticka, 57, of Hillsboro, Oregon.

Sticka is one of millions of people benefiting from compounding—when pharmacists prepare drugs in doses, forms, and combinations not available from manufacturers. In this case, the standard prescription testosterone gel (AndroGel) is suitable only for men, delivering several times the daily dose that Sticka's doctor prescribed.

More than 30 million prescriptions are compounded each year, and they're a godsend for people with needs that off-the-shelf pharmaceuticals can't meet. But these drugs have recently come under attack. Critics are concerned that some compounders are acting like drug manufacturers, doctors, or both—but without the same safeguards. There's good reason to be worried: Compounded drugs are blamed for a host of serious side effects, including three recent deaths. Even if this is the first you've heard of compounding, you shouldn't feel immune to its potentially negative consequences. As the practice becomes more widespread (over the past decade, it's burgeoned into at least a $5 billion business), it has the potential to affect millions of people—including you.

Lifesaver or Risky Business?

All of the nearly 200,000 pharmacists in this country are licensed to compound, and about 5,000 make it a specialty. At their best, compounding pharmacists occupy a respected, time-honored position in the medical system. From modifying the strength of a medication to altering the form or flavor so it's easier to swallow, they fill a vital need if you can't take commercial, one-size-fits-all drugs.

The problem is the changing nature of compounding. Traditionally, it involves a sacrosanct "triad relationship" between a patient with a special need (such as Sticka), a physician who writes her a prescription, and a pharmacist who tailors the drug. But lately some shady drug manufacturers are calling themselves compounders to get around the FDA's stringent oversight of pharmaceuticals. Even some corner-drugstore types—in an effort to drum up new business and boost profits—seem to be overstepping their bounds in a way that puts consumers at risk.

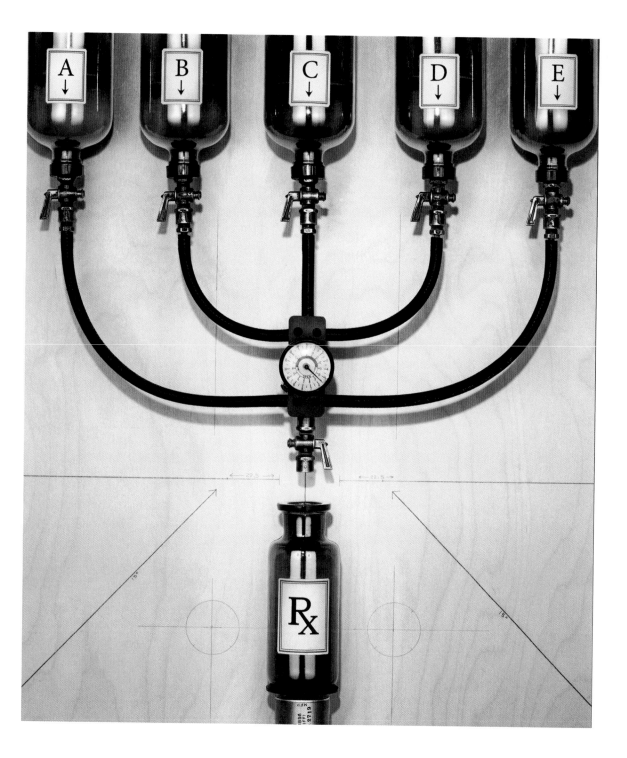

Compounding Goes Awry

Although compounders aren't supposed to make anything unless they receive a specific prescription, many are producing, stockpiling, and marketing large quantities of Rx drugs—creating what's being dubbed a shadow drug industry. However, unlike drugs made by the pharmaceutical industry, compounded medicines aren't regulated by the FDA. This lack of oversight is accepted when pharmacists make drugs for a single patient. But these large-scale compounders often employ poor manufacturing processes that can result in products without the required strength, quality, or purity—meaning an error could endanger many.

The Hormone Wars Heat Up

Bioidenticals have become the most visible targets of the FDA's recent actions on compounding. Last year it sent seven pharmacies warning letters charging that their Web sites made unsubstantiated claims about bioidenticals. It warned the pharmacies that they shouldn't be compounding any prescriptions containing estriol, which is a weak estrogen that's promoted as safer than other hormones but isn't a component of any FDA-approved product.

Compounders and their customers are fighting back. Last fall, in an orchestrated campaign, more than 25,000 patients, pharmacists, and physicians called their legislators to ask them to preserve their right to compounded medications, particularly bioidenticals, and to pass legislation to reverse the FDA's position on estriol.

"If something has worked all these years, why stop it?" asks Carol Pride, 62, of Augusta, Georgia, whose compounded hormonal formula was switched to the stronger estradiol after the FDA crackdown on estriol. "This is government interference."

Compounding proponents accuse the FDA of caving in to complaints by Wyeth Pharmaceuticals, the makers of Prempro, the estrogen-progestin combo deemed risky in the Women's Health Initiative study. But many independent groups, including the National Women's Health Network, supported Wyeth's request for greater regulation. For now, legislation demanding that the FDA reverse its estriol position is pending.

This worst-case scenario happened to Margrit Long of Portland, Oregon, who sought relief from chronic back pain. Her doctor suggested injections of colchicine, a drug used in pill form to treat gout, and prescribed off-label in injection form for back pain. The doctor got the medication from ApothéCure, a Dallas pharmacy that promotes its compounded injectables. The strong anti-inflammatory action of the shots seemed to help with Long's pain for several years—until March 2007, when an injection killed her. The problem: a measurement error by the person mixing the prescription, which meant that Long and at least two others were fatally injected with eight times the intended amount of colchicine. ApothéCure ultimately recalled more than 3,500 vials of the drug that had been distributed nationwide.

Precisely how many other compounding errors there are isn't known. That's because—unlike commercial drug manufacturers—pharmacies in most states aren't required to report adverse events associated with compounded drugs to the FDA or state pharmacy boards. But the one state that tests random samples of drugs has uncovered problems. When Missouri's board of pharmacy spot-checked compounded prescriptions in 2007, 51 of 213 prescriptions tested were more than 10 percent off in the dose of active ingredients, one had only one-fifth of the amount needed, and another had $4^1/_2$ times the prescribed dose.

Horror stories like Long's aren't the exclusive domain of large-scale compounders: Local compounding pharmacists can be overconfident in their ability to make what patients and physicians need. In 2001, Doc's Pharmacy in Walnut Creek, California, began compounding a steroid that the manufacturer had temporarily stopped making. But the reputable pharmacy was unable to create a sterile compound, and within a few months, three people treated with the contaminated injections died of meningitis. This outcome shouldn't be that surprising, considering that just one in five schools of pharmacy offers a special course on compounding sterile medications. Only 13 percent of pharmacy-school deans felt that their students graduated with adequate training in compounding sterile preparations, according to a 2005 survey. Yet all pharmacists are licensed to compound.

Pharmacists as Physicians?

Some compounders veer toward practicing medicine themselves, dispensing advice directly to women on the best drug for their ills. This is especially true when it comes to "bioidenticals." These prescription hormones, frequently used to treat perimenopausal discomfort, are synthesized to be molecularly identical to specific human hormones. It's okay for compounders to make up prescriptions for various combinations of hormones, but compounders frequently promote bioidenticals as natural, risk free, and able to prevent or cure a host of medical conditions. The truth: Bioidenticals are created in a laboratory, often through the manipulation of plant hormones, and there's no proof that they have fewer or different risks than other hormones or offer any specific health benefits.

But that's not what many women hear. At some pharmacies, you can go to a lecture on the benefits of bioidenticals, schedule an individual consultation to review your symptoms, take hormone tests that the pharmacist analyzes, and have a customized bioidentical hormone prescription recommended and sent to your physician's office for a signature. If your doctor's not amenable, the pharmacy helps you find a physician who is.

Experts, including the FDA, strongly object to how bioidenticals are being promoted, especially because many of these same claims were made—and proved wrong—about commercial estrogen products. Indeed, in a 2001 study of 664 post-

COMPOUNDED DRUGS: A GUIDE TO SAFETY

SCREEN YOUR PHARMACIST

Ask your physician to recommend a compounder, and ask the pharmacist whether she regularly compounds the drug you need. If the answer is no, look for another who does.

Confirm that a compounder is licensed and in good standing before ordering. If it's an out-of-state pharmacy, check the Web sites of the state board of pharmacy in your state and theirs, advises Carmen Catizone, PharmD, executive director of the National Association of Boards of Pharmacy. Web sites and e-mail addresses for all state boards are available at www.nabp.net.

Check whether an Internet pharmacy is recommended at www.nabp.net. Just say no if it's one of the "not recommended sites" known to be out of compliance with federal and state laws and patient safety standards.

Find out if the pharmacy is accredited by the Pharmacy Compounding Accreditation Board, which compounders established to certify pharmacies. (Its Web site, www.pcab.org, has a map of accredited pharmacies.) It's neither an absolute necessity nor a guarantee of quality, but it's one indicator that the company takes compounding seriously and practices quality control.

RESEARCH THE DRUGS

Ask whether the same drug is available without compounding. Some pharmacists increase profits by compounding a prescription when a very similar manufactured product is available.

menopausal women, when the estradiol used in many compounded formulas was tested for its ability to prevent a repeat stroke, women who took the hormone had no fewer heart attacks or strokes—and their strokes were more severe and more often fatal.

"Compounding can be a fine way to get low doses of hormone therapy. But hormones don't magically become safer because they're compounded. They just lose their warning labels," says Adriane Fugh-Berman, MD, an associate professor in the complementary and alternative medicine program at Georgetown University Medical Center in Washington, DC.

"Compounding Saved My Life"

Negative publicity hasn't shaken Ottilie Ruh's confidence in compounding. After developing a severe corn allergy at 43, Ruh, of Salem, Oregon, became dependent on compounding because nearly all drugs contain corn as an inactive filler. It's more

Check with your doctor if your drug label says it was compounded and you didn't expect it to be. All compounded medication must be labeled as such.

Think twice if you're prescribed a compounded version of a drug that's no longer on the market. Ask why and heed any safety concerns.

Think three times before getting a compounded drug that's in timed-release form or designed to be inhaled or injected. In general, bacteria and other impurities are most dangerous when injected or inhaled. It's tricky to produce timed-release capsules so that the drug is delivered at an even pace.

MINIMIZE SIDE EFFECTS

Look up your drugs. Compounded medications may come without warning labels or information about side effects, but that doesn't make them risk free. Talk with your doctor about precautions before having your prescription filled. Ask the pharmacist to show you the patient labeling for a commercial product with the same active ingredient, or look up standard warnings yourself by checking the active ingredient on Web sites such as www.rxlist.com.

Notify your doctor and pharmacist if your condition worsens while you're using compounded meds. Make sure the product isn't the problem before you refill or up your dose.

Use, store, and discard medication correctly. (Ask your doctor or pharmacist how.) A drug compounded into a liquid form, for example, might have a very short shelf life and require refrigeration.

expensive to have her medications—antibiotics, steroids, and aspirin—made into corn-free formulations. But the extra cost is worth it, says Ruh, who insists, "I'd be dead without compounded drugs."

Testimonials like this are what make compounding so much more rewarding than traditional retail pharmacy, practitioners maintain. "There are bad eggs in every industry, but ours as a whole is a very caring profession," says Dana Reed-Kane, PharmD, co-owner of Reed Pharmacy in Tucson. "Our passion is helping people with unique needs."

But for every positive story about compounding, there seems to be another casting it in a negative light. In one egregious example of what compounders will do to increase profits, some pharmacies have even taken it upon themselves to change doctors' commercial prescriptions (often for more expensive brand-name drugs) to compounded mixtures (which can be produced less expensively)—frequently on the sly and sometimes to dangerous effect.

In 1996, Margaret Davis's lifelong lung problems—which she controlled by breathing two commercial medications through a nebulizer—mysteriously veered out of control. Turned out that a company, advertising the convenience of having a portable breathing machine delivered along with her meds, had faxed her doctors a form to initiate payment for the machine. They signed, unaware that hidden in the fine print was a blanket authorization for compounding. The pharmacy began substituting a compounded version of her primary medication for the real thing, adding a third that was never prescribed and mixing them all together in a way that made the drugs impossible to use correctly. Once the problem was discovered and Davis began breathing in her prescribed formula, her disease came back under control.

Who's in Charge?

All compounding pharmacies are licensed and regulated by state boards of pharmacy, which have little money for enforcement.

"Rigorous oversight is really a myth in most states," says Larry D. Sasich, PharmD, chairman of the department of pharmacy practice at the Lake Erie College of Osteopathic Medicine in Pennsylvania. "Inspections are few and far between."

Although the FDA regulates the safety and effectiveness of manufactured drugs, it allowed the traditional compounding of individual prescriptions—permitting compounders to make up enough products in advance to fill prescriptions that they routinely receive. But the FDA is stepping in now that compounding seems to have morphed into disguised manufacturing.

Last summer, for instance, it sent a

stern warning letter to the Medi-Stat pharmacy in Mobile, Alabama. On its Web site, Medi-Stat promoted its own line of pain-relieving creams that contained combinations of ingredients not proven to be safe or to work. According to the letter, it produced large volumes of the creams and employed sales reps to visit physicians' offices with promotional materials, samples, and preprinted prescription pads for the products—in short, acting like an FDA-regulated pharmaceutical company. The only difference: None of Medi-Stat's formulations are FDA approved or produced under the safe manufacturing guidelines that drug companies must follow.

As the FDA tries to take more control, compounders are stepping up self-regulation and suing to stay regulated by the states. The whole issue isn't likely to be sorted out for years. Until it is, it's essential that you make every effort to protect yourself when buying a compounded drug (see "Compounded Drugs: A Guide to Safety" on page 40). In a lesson that cost Margrit Long and others their lives, it's clearly an area where medicine has the opportunity to do great harm as well as great good.

EAT

"You are what you eat" is even

PART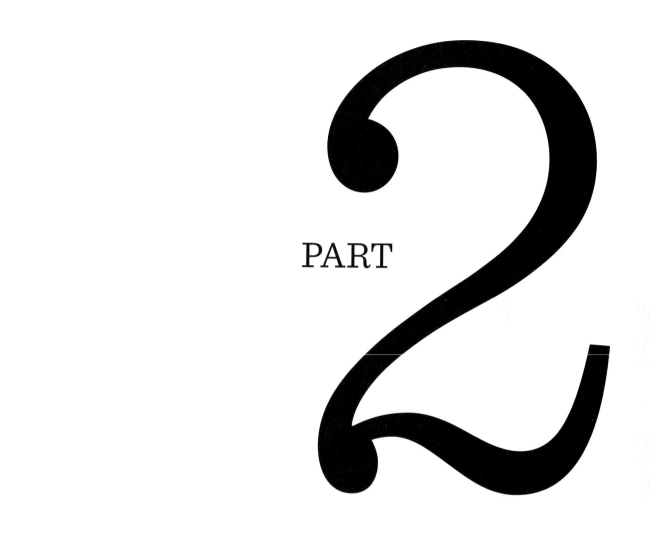

2

RIGHT

more true when you have diabetes.

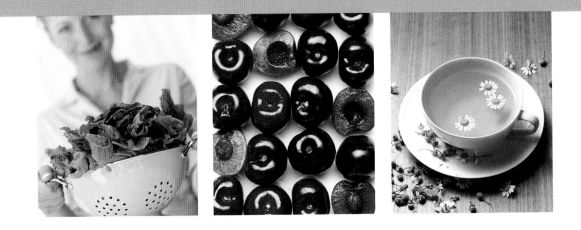

NUTRITION
Medical Breakthroughs

Do you live to eat? Having diabetes shouldn't ruin your enjoyment of food. Instead, planning your meals, shopping for nutritious ingredients, and cooking healthy (and delicious) foods can enhance your love to eat. **Now you can eat to live!**

EAT TO BEAT DIABETES

What you eat (and don't) might play a major role in your risk of developing type 2 diabetes, according to a new study from researchers at Tulane University and the Harvard School of Public Health who tracked the eating habits of more than 71,000 women for 18 years. Here's how to prevent the disease, based on their research.

Add: Leafy greens. For every additional serving of spinach, kale, or Swiss chard you eat, you might lessen your risk by as much as 9 percent.

Add: Whole fruit. For every three servings, you might slash your diabetes risk by up to 18 percent.

Avoid: Juice. Consuming one serving a day might raise your odds by nearly 18 percent. Some varieties are rich in antioxidants, but if you're at risk of diabetes, consider trading your daily glass of juice for whole fruit.

Avoid: Sugar. Although eating sugar doesn't cause diabetes in the same smoking gun way that cigarettes cause cancer, research shows that sugar may play a part, and it's smart to limit your intake. First, consuming too much sugar can lead to weight gain, and being overweight does increase your risk of developing type 2 diabetes. Emerging research also suggests that excess sugar intake can increase diabetes risk regardless of weight. A landmark study in the *Journal of the American Medical*

Nut	Benefits in Every Bite
Almonds	One ounce has as many heart-healthy polyphenols as a cup of green tea and ½ cup of steamed broccoli combined; shown to help lower LDL cholesterol.
Hazelnuts	Rich in arginine, which is an amino acid that can relax blood vessels and may lower blood pressure, hazelnuts also have high levels of vitamin E, folate, and B vitamins.
Peanuts	Packed with protein, fiber, healthy fats, and a host of other nutrients, peanuts—if eaten regularly—are linked with lower weight and decreased risk of diabetes.
Pecans	Highest overall concentration of disease-fighting antioxidants among all nuts; 1 ounce contains 10 percent of your daily value for fiber.
Pistachios	A daily serving or two may decrease LDL levels by 9 to 12 percent, according to a recent Pennsylvania State University study.

Association found that women nearly doubled their diabetes risk when they increased the number of sweetened drinks they had from one or less a week to one or more per day over an 8-year period. Rapidly absorbed sugars—such as those in colas—might damage the pancreas cells that secrete insulin, according to study author Frank B. Hu, MD, PhD, a professor of nutrition and epidemiology at the Harvard School of Public Health.

▓ GO A LITTLE NUTS

Eating $1^1/_2$ ounces (a couple of handfuls) of tree nuts as a daily snack can reduce your risk of diabetes and heart disease, according to USDA researchers. But only 34 percent of people eat any nuts at all, reports a government survey. See the box on page 47 for five types worth trying for good health and great taste.

▓ EAT AN APPLE A DAY

This unassuming superfruit boasts a bevy of health benefits, and new science shows that this supermarket staple packs a powerful disease-fighting punch. Its pectin and polyphenols may help prevent colon cancer, suggests a study published in *Nutrition*. And Cornell University scientists discovered that feeding mice the equivalent of one apple daily reduced breast cancer tumor growth by 24 percent. Plus, apple-eating adults have a 27 percent lower risk of metabolic syndrome, according to researchers.

TURN A LITTLE BLUE

Grab some wild blueberries when you stock up on frozen foods. Researchers at Cornell University tested 25 fruits for antioxidant activity and found that tangy-sweet wild blueberries (which are smaller than their cultivated cousins) packed the most absorbable antioxidants. Their levels exceeded those of nutrient-rich pomegranates and grapes.

Buy: Frozen brands like Dole and Wyman's of Maine.

Try: Tossing them into salads or mixing with $1/_2$ cup of low-fat ricotta and a drizzle of honey.

HARNESS THE POWER OF PITS

For a hefty helping of disease-fighting antioxidants, sink your teeth into a juicy, portable peach, nectarine, or plum. Each stone fruit—so called because of the hard pit surrounding a seed—has potent antioxidants. According to scientists at Texas AgriLife Research, just one plum contains at least the same levels of phytonutrients and antioxidants as at least 1 cup of blueberries.

Because stone fruits fit in the palm of your hand, it's easy to get your antioxidants on the run. When they're in season, in spring, they'll taste fresh and cost less.

▓ KEEP PRODUCE FRESH LONGER

For the best deals on summer's bounty, head to your local farmers' market. You'll save big on in-season fruits and veggies and find just-picked crops that are more nutritious than their store-bought counterparts. The problem: With the abundance comes spoilage. *Prevention* spoke with Marita Cantwell, PhD, a postharvest specialist at the University of California, Davis, and got her simple—and surprising—storage secrets for stretching the life of perishable produce. Here are her store-longer do's and don'ts.

Watermelon

Do: Ripen on your countertop for about a week, which nearly doubles the melon's lycopene and beta-carotene levels, according to a USDA study. Pop it in the fridge a day before eating.

Don't: Store it near other fruits; watermelon is easily damaged by ethylene, a gas released by fruits that speeds up deterioration.

Grapes

Do: Store in their original ventilated plastic bag, remove bruised or damaged fruit, and wrap the rest in paper towels to absorb excess moisture that promotes mold growth.

Don't: Wash until right before eating; doing so in advance encourages mold development.

Fresh Herbs

Do: Wrap in paper towels to absorb moisture, and place in a plastic bag in the crisper drawer.

Don't: Refrigerate basil, which is damaged by the cold; stand it in water on a sunny windowsill.

Tomatoes

Do: Store cherry and grape tomatoes in their original containers in the refrigerator. Ripen large varieties on the counter. Cold temperatures halt color, flavor, and nutrient development. Once they're bright red, store them in the fridge.

Don't: Place ripe tomatoes near vegetables because tomatoes give off ethylene.

Berries

Do: Store in their original clamshell containers, which increase ventilation. Remove bruised or moldy berries from the batch; they'll speed up decay among the rest.

Don't: Wash berries prior to storage for the same reason as grapes.

Leafy Greens

Do: Pat them dry before storing because excess moisture contributes to decay. Wrap in paper towels, place in a plastic bag, and store in the crisper.

Don't: Keep them near ethylene-emitting fruits such as tomatoes.

▦ SPICE UP YOUR LIFE

A touch of spice might be just what you need to minimize the damage of aging—and even help offset the impact of diabetes. New research from the University of Georgia found that antioxidant-rich herbs and spices can block the formation of harmful compounds that are associated with aging and might inhibit tissue damage caused by high levels of blood sugar.

A little spice goes quite a long way because the antioxidants are extremely

The percentage you can lower your risk of heart disease by leading a healthy lifestyle, according to the National Heart, Lung, and Blood Institute:

82

The grams of fiber in 1 cup of frozen wild blueberries:

6

concentrated, says study coauthor James Hargrove, PhD. Here are the top seven picks studied and how to include them in your diet.

Ground Cloves

Try it: In cake or biscuit dough for an added layer of spicy sweetness.

Ground Jamaican Allspice

Try it: In lean ground beef to add an unexpected twist to hamburgers or meat loaf.

Sage

Try it: In your favorite tomato sauce recipe.

Marjoram

Try it: Steeped in hot water for an herbal tea.

Ground Cinnamon

Try it: On whole wheat toast drizzled with honey.

Ground Oregano

Try it: On top of homemade garlic bread or pizza.

Thyme

Try it: In scrambled eggs for a fragrant flavor boost.

▥ SIP FOR BETTER BLOOD SUGAR

Enjoying a cup of chamomile tea is more than a soothing nighttime ritual. The herb may help rein in blood sugar fluctuations and prevent the ravages of type 2 diabetes, according to a recent study.

When researchers fed chamomile tea to rats with diabetes, the animals had significant decreases in blood sugar and lower levels of compounds that can cause diabetes complications. Although more research

is needed, people with diabetes might reap the same benefits from sipping chamomile daily, according to the scientists.

▥ DRINK TO YOUR HEART'S CONTENT

People at high risk for heart disease who drink a mixture of no-sugar-added cocoa powder and fat-free milk twice a day have lower levels of inflammation—an indicator of atherosclerosis—compared with those who drink only milk, according to a Spanish study. Researchers believe the high concentration of polyphenols in cocoa powder works as a natural anti-inflammatory. Drink chocolate milk or eat polyphenol-rich foods—such as dark chocolate, grapes, and berries—daily.

▥ CHOOSE A BETTER OMEGA-3

The best omega-3s might be farther down the food chain. Two studies (one manufacturer funded) showed that fatty acid–rich krill oil—extracted from a tiny, shrimplike sea creature—more effectively reduces blood sugar, LDL cholesterol, and even PMS symptoms than fish oil. Both oil supplements are reliably contaminant free, but there are still too few studies to know how krill oil truly stacks up, especially for heart health, according to Cynthia Sass, MPH, RD.

Plus, krill oil might pose two dangers: one to people with shellfish allergies, Sass says, and the other to your wallet. It can cost several times more than fish oil supplements because krill are in shorter supply.

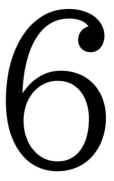

Beat Diabetes
WITH FOOD

Prevention asked a top certified diabetes educator the tough questions about eating right with diabetes. Her replies will help you **eat to live, and live to eat—despite diabetes.**

For people living with type 2 diabetes, dozens of questions can arise. With insights on some of the most common questions her clients face, Ann Fittante, MS, RD, a registered dietitian and certified diabetes educator at the Joslin Diabetes Center education affiliate at Swedish Medical Center in Seattle, offers answers.

Of course, before undertaking any weight-loss program or change in your eating plan, talk with your personal physician, dietitian, or certified diabetes educator to make sure it's the right decision for you.

How can I tell if a specific food raises my blood glucose? The best way to determine the effects of food on blood glucose levels is to monitor your glucose before the meal and then either 1, 2, or 3 hours after the meal. I prefer using the 2-hour test. Blood glucose targets for most people with diabetes are:

- 90–130 mg/dL before meals
- Less than 180 mg/dL 1 hour after meals
- Less than 160 mg/dL 2 hours after meals
- Less than 140 mg/dL 3 hours after meals

For example, if your glucose level before eating chicken, 1 cup of rice, and 1 cup of broccoli is 120 mg/dL and 2 hours later it is 150 mg/dL, you know the portion sizes in that meal (more specifically the carbohydrate amounts) are appropriate for you. If, however, before a meal of pasta, bread, and chocolate cake your glucose level is 120 mg/dL and 2 hours later it is 250 mg/dL, you know the carbohydrate amounts of that meal are too high for you.

I always thought that regular sugar was forbidden for those with diabetes, but lately I've been seeing recipes that call for sugar. Is it okay to eat sugar? Yes, it's okay to eat sugar. Sugar is a carbohydrate and does not raise glucose levels more than other sources of carbohydrate. Because foods that contain quite a bit of sugar and fat (like desserts) are sources of empty calories, it is best to limit the amount. One teaspoon of sugar, honey, jam, or jelly has 4 grams of carbohydrate, which will not raise glucose levels very much. I recommend limiting sugar to 1 to 2 teaspoons at one time and limiting desserts to 30 grams or fewer of carbohydrate. If you are going to eat a high-carbohydrate dessert like cake or pie, combining it with a lower-carbohydrate meal like fish and non-starchy vegetables will keep glucose levels in a better range than if you ate it with a higher-carbohydrate meal such as pasta.

Should I stick to the same foods every day? Eating a variety of foods ensures a healthier diet. But I know many people with diabetes tend to stick to the same foods since they can better predict how these foods will affect their glucose levels. Learning the carbohydrate amounts in new foods can help you decide the right portion sizes so that your glucose level stays on target. Eating seasonally is a good strategy for increasing variety. Fruits and vegetables taste much better and cost less when they are newly harvested.

Another strategy is to eat foods by the color of a rainbow. Choose red foods (red apples, red peppers), orange (carrots, winter squash), yellow (banana, yellow peppers), green (kiwifruit, spinach), blue (blueberries), and violet (eggplant, concord grapes). Aim for variety if possible

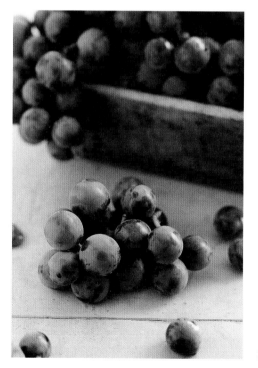

because you get different nutrients from different foods. Your diet is likely to be healthier.

Is broccoli some kind of magic food for diabetes? My blood glucose always tests normal after I eat it, no matter what other "bad" foods I have with the meal. I think broccoli is a magic food because it is packed with nutrients and fiber! I have not heard specifically that eating it seems to cause blood glucose levels to be lower, however. Most nonstarchy vegetables are very low in carbohydrate and have minimal impact on blood glucose levels. It may be that when you eat the "bad" food with broccoli, the entire meal is not very high in carbohydrate, and it is for that reason your blood glucose level is lower.

I heard alcohol lowers blood glucose levels. Is this true? It is true that alcohol can lower blood glucose levels in some people with diabetes. This is especially true if you are on a medication like insulin or certain pills for diabetes that can cause low blood glucose. To prevent low blood glucose if you drink, it is best to include a carbohydrate snack like whole grain crackers or popcorn or have the drink with a meal. Mixed drinks can increase blood glucose levels because the "mixer" is usually high in carbohydrates (sugar). Beer, wine, and hard liquor have minimal impact on blood glucose levels if consumed in small amounts. General recommendations for alcohol are to limit to one drink per day for women and two drinks per day for

A BAKER'S DOZEN INDULGENCES

When you're diagnosed with diabetes, the challenge of adapting the way you eat—especially at the beginning—can feel daunting.

For times like these, Ann Fittante, MS, RD, a registered dietitian and certified diabetes educator at the Joslin Diabetes Center education affiliate at Swedish Medical Center in Seattle, gives the green light to "indulgences" that are okay to eat once in a while (two or three times a month). Eating the amounts listed should not increase blood glucose levels significantly or ruin your weight loss efforts. Each "indulgence" is approximately 30 grams of carbohydrate and 250 calories or fewer.

- ½ cup regular ice cream (not gourmet or premium types, which are much higher in fat)
- 1 ounce milk, semisweet, or bittersweet chocolate
- 1 ounce snack chips
- ½ bag microwave popcorn
- 2 or 3 small cookies
- ¼ cup chocolate chips
- 8 chocolate kisses
- 3 cups kettle corn
- 1 small serving french fries
- 1 doughnut
- 1 small flavored latte, mocha, or frappuccino coffee drink
- 2 small "Halloween"-size candy bars
- 1 small cannoli

men. Remember, alcohol contributes excess calories and can make weight loss more difficult. One drink is approximately 80 to 150 calories.

Dried cereal seems to raise my blood glucose significantly. Why is that? Many dried cereals are very high in carbohydrate even though they may be high in beneficial fiber and have little or no sugar. The combination of a medium to large bowl (one to three servings) of cereal, fruit, and milk increases the carbohydrate content of the meal significantly. To see the effects of dried cereal on your blood glucose levels, test glucose levels before and 2 hours after eating. Remember the 2-hour blood glucose goal is 160 mg/dL or less. Hot cereals are less processed and tend not to raise glucose levels as much as dried cereals.

I heard fruit raises blood glucose levels. Is this true? Fruit is a carbohydrate and if eaten in large quantities can increase blood glucose levels. Fruit is high in fiber and important nutrients, as well as relatively low in calories, so you should eat fruit daily. A medium piece of fruit (like an apple, an orange, or 1 cup of grapes) is approximately 30 grams of carbohydrate and should not increase glucose levels too much. My general recommendation is to include one to three pieces of fruit per day, eating one piece at one time (spacing it out over the course of several meals). If fruit seems to be increasing your blood glucose level, include it with some protein or fat (cottage cheese or nuts), which may slow the absorption and prevent the glucose from increasing too much.

Will eating too much protein put a strain on my kidneys? If you already have kidney disease, eating too much protein may put more strain on your kidneys. For this reason, high-protein diets are discouraged. Limiting animal protein to 6 ounces per day is a good place to start if you already have kidney disease. Ask your physician or dietitian for more specific recommendations. If you do not have kidney disease, eating more protein probably won't negatively affect your kidneys; however, a more balanced meal plan approach (eating carbohydrate, protein, and healthy fat with meals) is still recommended for best nutrition.

Can I eat salt? Does it raise my blood glucose levels? Salt, or sodium chloride, does not raise blood glucose levels. If you have high blood pressure, kidney disease, or congestive heart failure, limiting sodium in your diet is very important. Too much sodium can also cause fluid retention. *Prevention* recommends limiting sodium to 2,300 milligrams per day for optimal health. If you have high blood pressure,

kidney disease, or congestive heart failure, limiting sodium further to 1,500 to 2,000 milligrams per day may be beneficial. Avoiding processed food products that typically contain high amounts of sodium can eliminate a great deal of sodium from your diet.

My trainer wants me to eat a snack before exercise. What should I be eating? If the reason your trainer wants you to snack before exercise is to prevent low blood glucose, first consider if you are at risk for low blood glucose (hypoglycemia). People who are not on medication for diabetes are not at risk for hypoglycemia. Some medications for diabetes also do not cause hypoglycemia, and therefore having a snack may not be necessary. Consuming snacks may add unnecessary calories, especially if weight loss is your goal. However, if it's been several hours since your last meal, having a snack before exercise may provide extra fuel and help maximize your workout. I suggest 15 to 30 grams of carbohydrate and fewer than 200 calories (for example., fruit and 6 nuts; $^1/_2$ serving crackers and 1 teaspoon peanut butter; or 1 cup of plain, low-fat yogurt with $^1/_2$ cup berries).

How do protein and fat affect blood glucose levels? Protein and fat have minimal effects on blood glucose levels. They both slow absorption of carbohydrate. As the carbohydrate, such as bread, in a meal is digested and transformed into blood

(continued on page 58)

GO—SLOW—WHOA FOODS

Post this chart on your refrigerator or take it along when you shop for food.

Go foods: Eat almost anytime. Nutrient-dense foods that are the highest in quality and the least processed. Low in fat, sugar, sodium, and calories. In the plant groups, they are highest in fiber.

Slow foods: Eat sometimes, at most several times a week. These foods are more processed and may be high in fat, added sugar, sodium, and calories.

Whoa foods: Eat only once in a while or for special treats, about three times a month. These are low-nutrient foods that may be highly processed and may contain unnecessary additives. Highest in fat, sugar, and sodium. In the plant food groups, they are lowest in fiber.

VEGETABLES

Go: Fresh, plain frozen, or low-sodium canned vegetables with no added fat and sauces; homemade oven-baked "french fries"

Slow: All vegetables cooked with moderate amounts of healthy unsaturated fats (such as olive and canola oils) and low-fat tomato sauces

Whoa: French fried potatoes, hash browns, or other fried potatoes; other deep-fried vegetables; frozen vegetables in cheese or other high-fat sauces

FRUITS

Go: All fresh, frozen, dried, and canned (in juice) fruits

Slow: Fruits canned in light syrup

Whoa: Fruits canned in heavy syrup

BREADS AND CEREALS

Go: Whole grain types of the following: breads, pitas, crackers, tortillas, pasta, brown rice, waffles; steel-cut oats and other hot breakfast cereals; cooked bulgur, barley, and quinoa; homemade low-fat whole grain muffins; homemade whole grain French toast and pancakes

Slow: Refined-flour products or other refined grains: bread, white rice, pasta, French toast, biscuits, and pancakes

Whoa: High-fat, refined-flour products: commercially prepared croissants, muffins, doughnuts, sweet rolls, and crackers made with trans fats; sweetened breakfast cereals

MILK AND DAIRY PRODUCTS

Go: Fat-free or 1% milk; fat-free or low-fat plain yogurt; part skim, reduced-fat, and fat-free cheese; 1% or fat-free cottage cheese

Slow: 2% milk; cream cheese, goat, and feta cheese; small amounts of regular full-fat cheese such as American, Cheddar, Swiss, Monterey Jack, Colby, Parmesan (no more than 2 to 3 ounces per week)

Whoa: Whole milk; whole-milk yogurt; processed cheese spread

BEANS, SOY, FISH, POULTRY, MEATS, EGGS, AND NUTS

Go: All dried beans or canned beans, split peas, lentils, hummus; tofu; tuna canned in water; baked, broiled, steamed, or grilled fish and shellfish; chicken and turkey without skin; fat-trimmed beef and pork; extra-lean ground beef; eggs (limit four egg yolks per week); Canadian bacon; all-natural peanut butter; 1 ounce nuts (three or four times per week)

Slow: Frozen veggie burgers; lean ground beef, broiled hamburgers; ham; chicken and turkey with skin; low-fat hot dogs; tuna canned in oil

Whoa: Fried fish and shellfish; fried chicken, chicken nuggets; untrimmed beef and pork; regular ground beef; fried hamburgers; ribs; bacon; hot dogs, delicatessen meats, pepperoni, sausage

SWEETS AND SNACKS

Go: Popcorn made with healthy fats, whole-grain tortilla chips, baked chips, whole grain crackers and crispbreads, homemade muffins or quick breads made with healthy fats and whole grain flour; homemade desserts with quality ingredients; dark chocolate; ice milk bars and low-fat ice cream; boxed gingersnaps, animal crackers, graham crackers

(Though some of these "go" choices are lower in fat and calories, all sweets and snacks need to be limited in order not to exceed one's daily calorie requirements.)

Slow: Frozen fruit juice bars; low-fat frozen yogurt or sorbet; packaged fig bars, pretzels, lowfat microwave popcorn

Whoa: Commercial cookies and cakes; pies; cheesecake; ice cream; candy; chips; microwave popcorn

FAT

Go: Olive, canola, and other unsaturated vegetable oils; unsaturated oil-based salad dressing, mayonnaise, and low-fat mayonnaise; low-fat sour cream; 1 ounce nuts (three or four times per week); pesto; 1/8 avocado,

Slow: Tartar sauce; sour cream; olives; trans-fat free spread; butter

Whoa: Margarine, solid vegetable shortening, lard; salt pork; gravy; regular creamy salad dressing; cheese sauce; cream sauce; cream cheese dips

BEVERAGES

Go: Water, fat-free milk, 1% milk, club soda or seltzer water, mineral water, unsweetened iced tea with lemon, herbal tea

Slow: 2% milk, wine, beer, hard liquor, sports drinks

Whoa: Whole milk; regular and diet soda; sweetened iced teas and lemonade; fruit drinks and fruit juice, diet iced teas, and diet lemonade

Source: Adapted from the National Heart, Lung, and Blood Institute (NHLBI). Published by the US Department of Health and Human Services; Public Health Service; National Institutes of Health; and the National Heart, Lung, and Blood Institute, Bethesda, Maryland.

glucose, the protein and fat, such as turkey and mayonnaise, in the meal slow the absorption of the glucose and prevent spikes in blood glucose levels. In some situations, very high-fat meals can slow down the absorption process too much, keeping blood glucose levels higher than desired for a longer period of time. Generally, the highest blood glucose level is approximately 1 hour after eating, and by 2 hours it should come back down (remember the target is less than 160 mg/dL). A very fatty meal of fish and chips may cause blood glucose levels to stay higher for 3 to 5 hours after eating because the fat in the meal slows absorption and keeps the glucose levels higher for a longer period of time. In situations like this, decreasing the fat in the meal will not only decrease extra calories but will also help bring your glucose levels back to target sooner. Fried fish and a salad or baked fish with fries would be a better balance. Baked fish with salad and a small baked potato is the best choice.

When my blood glucose level drops too low, what should I be eating to bring it back up? Symptoms of hypoglycemia (low blood glucose) include feeling shaky, sweaty, and dizzy, and being irritable, lightheaded, or very hungry. This can happen if blood glucose levels drop below 80 mg/dL. To bring blood glucose levels back up to normal as quickly as possible, have 15 grams of carbohydrate, like $1/_2$ cup juice, 1 tablespoon of honey, a small fruit,

2 tablespoons of raisins, or 3 glucose tablets.

Wait 15 minutes and retest. If blood glucose levels are not above 80 mg/dL, have another 15 grams of carbohydrate. Once blood glucose levels are above 80 mg/dL, you can eat a meal or have another carbohydrate/protein snack (such as toast with peanut butter) to sustain you until your next meal. Avoid treating hypoglycemia with carbohydrates that have added fat, like chocolate, granola bars, or cookies. These foods do not work quickly enough to bring your glucose levels back to normal.

I had a cold last week and my blood glucose levels went up to 200 mg/dL, and I was barely eating anything. Is this normal? Yes, it's very normal for blood glucose levels to increase when you are sick. Being sick stresses the body. When you are sick, you should continue monitoring your glucose levels. You may need to increase the frequency of testing to two to four times per day if your numbers are high. It's important to continue taking your diabetes medications when you are sick even if you are not eating very much. If blood glucose levels are 300 mg/dL or higher, call your doctor.

Can a person with diabetes ever get off diabetes medications? Yes, it is possible for some people with type 2 diabetes to either need less diabetes medication or get off it altogether with lifestyle changes. Typically, those people who no longer need their diabetes medications are those who lose weight if they are overweight and those who improve their fitness by exercising regularly.

Although some people strive to get off their diabetes medicines, it is not a sign of failure if that does not happen. Sometimes the body doesn't cooperate, and the amount of insulin your pancreas makes decreases and medications are necessary. It is important to remember that good blood glucose control is the goal whether it is controlled by diet, exercise, medication, or a combination of the three.

Are there vitamin/mineral supplements I should be taking? My overall recommendation is to try to obtain the nutrients you need through a balanced eating plan. However, taking a multivitamin for the added insurance of obtaining necessary nutrients is a good idea. If you are not getting three servings of a high-calcium food (milk, yogurt, cheese, dried fish, sardines, fortified soymilk), consider taking a calcium supplement with vitamin D in addition to the multivitamin. (The goal is 1,000 to 1,200 milligrams of calcium per day and 400 to 600 IU of vitamin D.) Deficiencies in minerals such as chromium, magnesium, and potassium may cause higher blood glucose levels in some people with diabetes. These nutrients can be obtained through both diet and a multivitamin supplement. Additional supplementation should not be necessary. There

has been interest in antioxidant supplementation in people with diabetes. Currently the recommendation is to obtain antioxidants through diet (fruits, veggies, whole grains).

My dietitian gave me a meal plan with recommended percentages of carbohydrate, protein, and fat, but I don't know how to translate those values into actual meals. Any advice? If you are unclear how to incorporate your dietitian's advice, I suggest calling him or her for clarification. Having a sample meal plan based on the recommendations will give you a better idea of how to translate the guidelines into actual meals. Using a healthy plate method is another meal plan approach.

With the plate method, fill half of your plate with vegetables, one-quarter of your plate with carbohydrate (rice, bread, pasta, fruit, milk), and one-quarter of your plate with protein and fat (meat, chicken, fish). If you don't eat vegetables for breakfast, fill one-third of your plate with protein, one-third with carbohydrate, and one-third with healthy fat. This guideline proportions the amount of carbohydrate, protein, and fat that is appropriate for most people with diabetes.

At the pharmacy, I noticed special "diabetic foods" like energy bars and shakes that promise to help control my blood glucose levels. Do I need to buy these kinds of products to be healthy? No, you do not need to buy specialty foods marketed to people with diabetes. Many times the carbohydrate content is slightly lower but not significantly lower than the traditional food. A "diabetes" bar might have 25 grams of carbohydrate compared to a regular granola bar with 30 grams of carbohydrate. Calories are the same. Fat content is the same, and in some cases the saturated fat (bad fat) is higher in the "diabetic" product. I've noticed that the specialty foods are more expensive and don't always taste as good. Check the ingredient list as well. Many times specialty foods have many more ingredients. They have been heavily fortified with vitamins and minerals. I believe the key to healthy eating is choosing foods that are less processed, and that means choosing foods with the fewest ingredients possible.

I've heard that diabetes is hereditary, and I'm worried my kids will develop the disease. How can I make sure they don't? Type 2 diabetes is hereditary and in the last several years becoming more prevalent in overweight children. Type 2 diabetes can be prevented or at least delayed until older age by maintaining a healthy weight, staying active, and eating healthfully. Eating right and being active is important for the entire family. Modeling these behaviors for your children helps them establish healthy lifestyle habits that they can maintain for life. Encourage the family to eat fruits and veggies daily; milk, yogurt, and cheese for calcium; lean meats; healthy fats; and snacks like popcorn, nuts, and peanut butter crackers. Limit the amount of soda, fast food, and unhealthy store-bought cookies and cake, chips, and doughnuts that your family consumes.

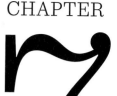

Feed What
AILS YOU

Diabetes plus the occasional headache or upset stomach can be just too much to take. Fortunately, **you can treat many common conditions with remedies straight from your kitchen.**

Many everyday foods contain nutrients and other properties that can ease common ills. From ginger for nausea to pineapple for hay fever, the following 17 kitchen cures will make you feel better fast!

Overstressed or Anxious?

Grab a banana.

Next time your buttons get pushed, reach for a banana, says Molly Kimball, RD, a certified specialist in sports dietetics with Ochsner's Elmwood Fitness Center in New Orleans. With only 105 calories and 14 grams of sugar, a medium banana fills you up, provides a mild blood sugar boost, and has 30 percent of the day's vitamin B6, which helps the brain produce mellowing serotonin, getting you through a crisis peacefully.

Plagued by High BP?

Toss back some raisins.

Sixty raisins—about a handful—contain 1 gram of fiber and 212 milligrams of potassium, both recommended in the Dietary Approaches to Stop Hypertension (DASH) diet. Numerous studies show that polyphenols in grape-derived foods such as raisins, wine, and juice are effective in maintaining cardiovascular health, including bringing down blood pressure.

Feeling Constipated or Gassy?

Reach for a yogurt.

One and a half cups of live-culture yogurt (high in gut-friendly bacteria) pushes food more efficiently through the gastrointestinal tract, says a 2002 study in *Alimentary Pharmacology & Therapeutics*. The beneficial bacteria also improve your gut's ability to digest beans and dairy lactose, which can cause gas, adds Kimball.

At Risk for Kidney Stones?

Load up on apricots.

Eight dried apricot halves have 2 grams of fiber, only 3 milligrams of sodium, and 325 milligrams of potassium—all of which help keep minerals from accumulating in urine and forming calcium oxalate stones, the most common type of kidney stones, says Christine Gerbstadt, MD, RD, an integrative nutritionist in private practice in Sarasota, Florida, and a spokesperson for the American Dietetic Association.

Got a Case of the Blues?

Open a can of tuna.

A 3-ounce serving of canned white tuna has about 800 milligrams of omega-3s, which research suggests may treat the kind of blues that leave you feeling low or anxious. The fatty acids in fish have been endorsed by the American Psychiatric Association as an effective part of depression treatment, says Elizabeth Somer, RD, author of *Eat Your Way to Happiness*.

For a seafood-free way to get happy, munch on a small bagel. The 37 grams of carbs will give you a dose of mood-boosting serotonin.

Feeling Nauseated?

Brew some ginger tea.

Dozens of studies reveal that ginger ($1/4$ teaspoon of powdered, $1/2$ to 1 teaspoon of minced gingerroot, or a cup of ginger tea) can ease nausea from motion sickness and pregnancy, says Gerbstadt. Researchers are unsure which oils and compounds in ginger suppress nausea, but it's safe and has none of the side effects (dry mouth, drowsiness) of OTC meds.

Got Tummy Troubles?

Pile on the basil.

Studies suggest that eugenol, a compound in basil, can keep your gut safe from pain, nausea, cramping, or diarrhea by killing off bacteria such as Salmonella and Listeria. Eugenol even has an antispasmodic property that can keep cramps at bay, says Mildred Mattfeldt-Beman, PhD, chair of the department of nutrition and dietetics at Saint Louis University. Use minced fresh basil in sauces or salads.

Coughing Too Much?

Swallow some buckwheat honey.

In a study at Pennsylvania State University, 2 teaspoons of thick, dark brown honey were more effective than OTC cough medicines at limiting the severity and frequency of a cough in children. Honey's antioxidants and antimicrobial properties may soothe inflamed throat tissues, says John La Puma, MD, director of Chef Clinic in California.

Given to Ulcers?

Cut up some cabbage.

A 2002 study at the Johns Hopkins School of Medicine found that sulforaphane, a powerful compound in cabbage, clobbers H. pylori (the bacteria that causes gastric and peptic ulcers) before it can get to your gut, and may even help inhibit the growth of gastric tumors. For only 34 calories a cup, cabbage provides 3 grams of fiber and 75 percent of the day's vitamin C.

Can't Sleep?

Munch on some turkey.

A 3-ounce serving of turkey has nearly all the tryptophan (an essential amino acid that helps the body produce serotonin and melatonin, hormones that regulate sleep) you need in a day, says La Puma. Studies show that people who suffer from insomnia are deficient in tryptophan.

Suffering from Hemorrhoids?

Fill up on figs.

The 3 grams of fiber in four dried figs helps create soft, regular stools that will keep hemorrhoids from returning, says Somer. Figs also provide about 5 percent of daily potassium and 10 percent of manganese.

Feeling Fatigued?

Down some OJ.

The fructose in a 4-ounce glass is a perfect pick-me-up, says Gerbstadt. Some studies suggest that vitamin C's ability to combat oxidative stress caused by free radicals may provide energy, and the vitamin plays a key role in metabolizing iron, which helps your body move energizing oxygen through your bloodstream, she adds.

Got a Yeast Infection?

Load up on garlic.

Garlic contains essential oils that can inhibit the growth of the Candida albicans fungus, the culprit in the pain, itch, and vaginal discharge of yeast infections, says Gerbstadt. Recent studies suggest that thyme, cloves, and even the essential oils from oranges are also effective fungicides, she adds. Include garlic in sauces, salad dressings, and marinades.

Irritated by Heartburn?

Drink chamomile tea.

"Chamomile can ease digestive inflammation, spasms, and gas," says Dale Bellisfield, RN, a clinical herbalist in New Jersey. Steep 2 teaspoons of the herb in 10 ounces of very hot water for 20 minutes, covering the cup to keep the essential oils in the water. You may have to drink the tea a few times a day for complete relief.

Can't Stop Sneezing?

Eat some pineapple.

Bromelain, an enzyme that's found in pineapple, can ease the symptoms of hay fever.

Prone to Headaches?

Bake a potato.

The 37 grams of carbs in a medium potato can ease a tension headache by increasing your levels of serotonin, as long as you keep the fat and protein below 2 grams.

Have High Cholesterol?

Grab a pear.

One medium pear has 5 grams of dietary fiber, most of it in the form of pectin, which helps flush out bad cholesterol, a risk factor in heart disease.

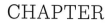

CHAPTER

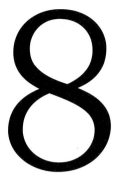

8

Go Power SHOPPING

Up the health ante of your grocery cart with our "good, better, and best" nutritional guide.

Your grocery cart is filled with good-for-you basics such as fresh produce, whole grains, and heart-smart oils. Now take your shopping list to the next level with even healthier picks.

"Eating a wide range of nutrient-dense foods gives you access to more vitamins, minerals, and other disease-fighting antioxidants," says David Grotto, RD, author of *101 Foods That Could Save Your Life!* Plus, having the same stuff day in and day out—even if it's great for you—qualifies as a rut, meaning you're missing out on new flavors, which help keep healthy eating fun. Our aisle-by-aisle guide to the good, better, and best supermarket superstars will help you make smart picks based on preference, availability, and budget. Upgrade your shopping list with these weight-busting, disease-fighting, energy-revving foods.

At the Meat Counter

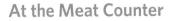

Good: Lean beef

Why: It's high in protein but lower in calories and saturated fat than other cuts of beef—and still brimming with B vitamins, which help your body turn food into energy. Cuts that have the word *loin* or *round* in their names (such as tenderloin or top round steak) are lower-fat choices. When you're buying ground beef, look for one that's at least 92 percent lean. (Beef labeled "80 percent lean" doesn't mean it has only 20 percent calories from fat. It's 20 percent fat by weight and has closer to 70 percent calories from fat—about 20 grams per 3½-ounce serving!)

Better: Organic beef

Why: The cattle were raised without hormones or antibiotics, substances that some experts worry may contribute to consumers' reproductive disorders and antibiotic resistance. Organic beef also makes a more environmentally friendly burger because it comes from cows fed only organic feed (which was grown without chemical pesticides). Just be sure the label says the word *organic* because natural beef isn't the same.

Best: Grass-fed beef

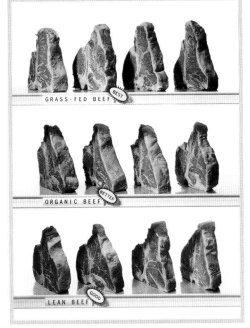

GRASS-FED BEEF · BEST

ORGANIC BEEF · BETTER

LEAN BEEF · GOOD

Why: It's pricier than regular beef, but the health perks make it worth the splurge. Compared with grain-fed beef, grass-fed packs twice the concentration of vitamin E, which is an antioxidant that protects cells from damage that can lead to chronic diseases. It's also high in CLAs, which are fatty acids that researchers link with weight loss. Plus, it's rich in heart-healthy omega-3 fatty acids, rivaling some fish. According to researchers from the University of California Cooperative Extension Service, feeding grass to cattle boosts the omega-3 content of beef by 60 percent. Because this type of beef tends to be lower in overall fat, it can be tough—so marinate it and use a meat thermometer to avoid overcooking.

In the Egg Section

Good: Packaged egg whites

Why: They're a low-calorie protein powerhouse, with no cholesterol or fat. In recipes, substitute the equivalent of two egg whites for each whole egg. Added bonus: Any egg-based dish makes an affordable alternative to pricier meat-based ones.

Better: Whole eggs

Why: The yolk is home to tons of nutrients, including choline, which is linked to lower rates of breast cancer. (One yolk has more than 25 percent of your daily needs.) It's also rich in antioxidants that may help prevent macular degeneration

and cataracts. Worried about the fat and cholesterol? Although people with heart disease should limit consumption of egg yolks to two a week, a recent study didn't find a connection between eating up to six eggs per week and increased rates of heart attack or stroke in healthy people.

Best: Omega-3–fortified eggs

Why: They have all the nutrients of regular eggs, plus up to 300 milligrams or so of the heart-protective fatty acids in each one. Many experts recommend 1,000 milligrams of DHA and EPA a day; however, because most people don't eat enough fish to meet this goal, these eggs offer another way to add omega-3s to your diet.

In the Dairy Case

Good: Fat-free milk

Why: It contains only traces of fat, while even 2 percent milk packs 3 grams of the artery-plugging saturated kind in every 8-ounce glass. Each cup of fat-free also supplies 76 milligrams more calcium than the same amount of whole milk does.

Better: Skim Plus

Why: It's as good for you as fat-free milk, with a richer taste. Skim Plus (also called skim deluxe or supreme) is fortified with extra milk protein, making it thicker, creamier tasting, and easier to transition to from whole or 2 percent.

Best: Organic fat-free milk

Why: A recent study from the United Kingdom found that organically raised cows produce milk with higher levels of antioxidants and fatty acids such as CLAs and omega-3s—thanks to all the grass and clover they consume. You'll pay more for organic milk, but because it's often ultrapasteurized (heated at higher temps and labeled UHT), it may last longer in your fridge.

On the Butter Shelf

Good: Trans-free margarine

Why: It's a wiser pick than butter because it doesn't contain any cholesterol and has much less saturated fat. It also doesn't pack the dangerous trans fats that many margarines do—the kind of fats that boost bad cholesterol and lower the good type. Some are even fortified with bone-building calcium or heart-healthy omega-3 fatty acids.

Better: Light trans-free margarine

Why: Your toast and baked potatoes will still get a buttery kick. But even if you use a whole tablespoon, you'll take in as few as 45 calories and 5 grams of fat.

Best: Margarine with added plant stanols and sterols

Why: You'll pay more for this margarine, but it's a powerful cholesterol fighter, thanks to plant stanols and sterols, which naturally reduce the amount of LDL cholesterol the body can absorb. In a study in the *American Journal of Cardiology*, eating 25 grams of margarine a day enriched with plant stanols and sterols lowered LDL cholesterol by 8 percent in 4 weeks.

In the Yogurt Section

Good: Low-fat flavored yogurt

Why: Cup for cup, yogurt has about 70 milligrams more calcium than milk, plus enough protein to make it a satisfying snack. It's rich in beneficial bacteria that can ward off tummy troubles and yeast infections. Look for lactobacillus (*L. acidophilus*) and/or bifidobacterium (*B. bifidum*) in the ingredients.

Better: Low-fat plain yogurt

Why: Despite the health benefits, some flavored varieties have a ton of added sweetener, such as sugar or high fructose corn syrup. For a healthier treat, pick plain and swirl in a spoonful of all-fruit spread. (You can also drizzle in honey for a bonus shot of antioxidants.)

Best: Greek yogurt

Why: "I love recommending Greek yogurt to clients," says Lara E. Metz, RD, a New York City–based nutritionist. "It has just as much calcium as regular yogurt and twice the protein, but it's richer and creamier." Be sure to choose the variety with zero percent fat to minimize calories.

At the Fish Counter

Good: Tilapia

Why: It's an affordable pick and a dieter's dream. Each 3-ounce serving contains only 110 calories and 2.5 grams of fat but a whopping 22 grams of fill-you-up protein. According to the FDA, tilapia has

CLICK FOR COUPONS

the lowest mercury level of all fish. Although other fish have more omega-3 fatty acids, tilapia is still a healthy choice at dinnertime.

Better: Halibut

Why: It boasts more omega-3s per serving than tilapia. In fact, a 5-ounce fillet packs your entire day's needs of EPA and DHA, fatty acids that can increase good HDL cholesterol and might also help prevent cognitive decline related to aging.

Best: Salmon

Why: It is one of the best sources of omega-3s you can find. Research has found that a healthy diet including fatty fish like salmon is linked to lower risk of heart disease, stroke, and diabetes. Wild has a slight edge over farm-raised because it may be lower in contaminants such as PCBs and dioxins—but both versions are equally nutritious. "Just remove the skin after cooking because that's where most of the contaminants are found," says Grotto.

In the Produce Section

Good: Romaine

Why: Rich in vitamins A and K, crunchy romaine makes a respectable base for any salad. Romaine also boasts more than eight times the vitamin C of iceberg lettuce.

Better: Watercress

Why: This peppery leaf adds not only a kick to salads but also a small dose of calcium. A study from the University of Ulster in the United Kingdom found that eating watercress daily is linked with reduced cellular DNA damage that may lead to cancer. If you find the flavor too strong, toss it with milder lettuces (say, Bibb or red leaf) or layer it with tomato on your turkey sandwich.

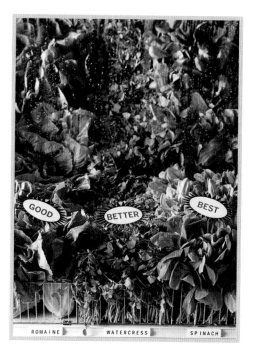

ROMAINE　　WATERCRESS　　SPINACH

Best: Spinach

Why: Spinach is rich in iron, which helps deliver oxygen to your cells to keep you alert and energized. And research from the Massachusetts Eye and Ear Infirmary links eating antioxidant-rich spinach with a lower risk of age-related macular degeneration.

In the Snack Aisle

Good: Popcorn

Why: It's a stealth whole grain, packing 3 grams of fiber and an entire serving of whole grains in each 3-cup, 90-calorie, air-popped bowl. That's why people who snack on it get two more servings of whole grains and 22 percent more fiber every day than people who don't, according to a recent study in the *Journal of the American Dietetic Association.*

Better: Peanuts

Why: With as much protein as $1/2$ cup of black beans, a handful of peanuts also contains 7 grams of heart-healthy monounsaturated fat. Women who ate peanuts and peanut butter at least five times a week had up to 27 percent less risk of developing type 2 diabetes, possibly because the healthy fats increase insulin sensitivity, according to a study from the Harvard School of Public Health. Because peanuts are easy to overeat, measure out your 1-ounce, 160-calorie portion (a small handful—about 40 nuts).

Best: Almonds

Why: "They're one of the most nutritious nuts around," says *Prevention* advisor David L. Katz, MD, director of the Yale-Griffin Prevention Research Center in Derby, Connecticut. Almonds are also the go-to snack when you're trying to drop weight. In one study, women who ate almonds had higher levels of the hunger-suppressing hormone cholecystokinin circulating in their systems. Another study found that a heart-healthy diet including almonds lowered LDL cholesterol as much as a statin drug did.

In the Dried-Fruit Bins

Good: Raisins

Why: They're an affordable and portable pick-me-up, ideal for stashing in your bag or desk drawer. Each little box contains one serving of fruit and nearly as much potassium as a small banana—but at 130 calories, they're a lighter pick than most energy bars. Researchers at the University of Illinois at Chicago College of Dentistry even debunked the myth that raisins stick to the teeth and cause cavities—they actually contain a natural compound that fights bacterial growth in the mouth.

Better: Dried apricots

Why: One-half cup contains all the virus-fighting vitamin A you need for the day, along with a big shot of potassium and the same amount of fiber as two slices of whole wheat bread. Sulfur

Save at the Supermarket

The average family of four throws out nearly 122 pounds of food per month. However, many common perishables, including these staples, remain perfectly safe as long as a week (or even a month) past their sell-by date when stored properly, which is 40°F or below.

Note: This is true provided that produce is purchased before the sell-by date. Always rely on your own senses—sight, smell, and touch—for signs of spoilage, and when in doubt, throw it out.

Food	Good For	Tip
Milk	1 week past sell-by date	Hit the dairy aisle right before checking out to minimize the amount of time milk is left unrefrigerated, and store it on a shelf pushed far back, where the air is coldest (closer to the door tends to be warmer).
Eggs	3–4 weeks past sell-by date	Store in their original container on a refrigerator shelf rather than on the door, where eggs are vulnerable to temperature fluctuations.
Hard cheese (once opened)	2–4 months past sell-by date	Wrap in moisture-proof plastic or foil; if the outside of hard cheese has visible mold, trim off the mold and a $1/2$-inch area of cheese below it.
Yogurt	10–14 days past sell-by date	Yogurt is best stored at around 39°F, an appropriate temp for your fridge. Don't be deterred by separation—simply stir and enjoy.
Lunchmeat (sealed)	3–5 days past sell-by date	Store meat in the meat compartment. It's specially designed to keep cool air in.

dioxide is often added to lock in color, but if it doesn't agree with your gut, look for an unsulfured kind (it's browner but just as healthy) or freeze-dried apricots, which are additive free.

Best: Dried figs

Why: With about one-third of your day's supply of fiber per $1/2$-cup serving, they pack more than any other dried fruit. Fiber helps you stay full, so figs are a powerful hunger suppressant. Each $1/2$ cup has as much calcium as $1/2$ ounce of cheese and contains phenols that may guard against heart disease and cancer, according to Grotto.

In the Condiments Aisle

Good: Low-fat creamy salad dressing

Why: If you prefer creamy dressings (such as ranch or blue cheese), this is a perfect way to add flavor to your favorite greens without drowning them in extra calories or fat.

Better: Full-fat oil-based dressing

Why: The fats in oils like canola and olive are healthier for you. They're a good source of vitamin E and help your body soak up all the vitamins in veggies. In one study, people absorbed more carotenoids from a salad with full-fat dressing than with reduced-fat dressing. (Those eating fat-free dressing absorbed just traces.) The calories add up fast, so measure out a 2-tablespoon portion.

Best: Olive oil and flavored vinegar

Why: With a do-it-yourself dressing, you don't have to worry about the quality of the ingredients. Mix 2 teaspoons of olive oil (or canola or flaxseed—they all contain higher amounts of heart-healthy monounsaturated fat) with flavored vinegar such as raspberry, then toss in any herbs you like.

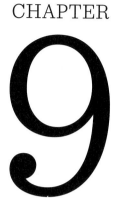
Unlock Your Body's Healing

POTENTIAL

A combo of foods, moves, and medical tests unlocks your body's healing potential. Reach your health goals—including sidestepping metabolic syndrome—faster with these 12 perfect unions.

Want more protection against skin cancer? Drink coffee before a workout. Trying to build muscle? Stretch between sets. Hoping to reduce your risk of stroke? Squeeze a little lemon into your green tea. Though seemingly random, these unusual combinations highlight the latest findings from the emerging practice that we call synergistic medicine, which pairs health-boosting strategies from fields as divergent as kinesiology, neuroscience, and dermatology—with truly outstanding results! We have rounded up the best dynamic duos for knocking out memory loss, fatigue, disease, weight gain, and more. Talk about power couples!

Avoid Metabolic Syndrome with the Mediterranean Diet + Nuts

A Mediterranean-style diet, rich in fruits, vegetables, beans, fish, olive oil, and grains, is associated with everything from weight loss to a reduced risk of Parkinson's and heart disease. Now new research shows that people with metabolic syndrome—which is a condition characterized by high blood sugar, cholesterol, and blood pressure and excess belly fat—can reduce these symptoms by adding an extra serving of mixed nuts to the healthful regimen.

In a large study, Spanish researchers instructed people at high risk of heart disease to follow the diet with slight variations. Among the group that added 30 grams of nuts, the incidence of metabolic syndrome decreased by about 14 percent within a year (as opposed to, say, a 6.7 percent decline in those who added a little more olive oil). Researchers believe that the fiber, potassium, magnesium, calcium, and omega-3 fatty acids in the nuts helped regulate insulin, blood pressure, and inflammation.

Healthy snack attack: Participants in the study ate about five walnuts, five hazelnuts, and five almonds daily. Kathy McManus, RD, director of the department of nutrition at Brigham and Women's Hospital in Boston, recommends eating the same amount (approximately 1 ounce) to take the edge off late-afternoon hunger. Sprinkle the mixture over Mediterranean-diet-friendly yogurt, hot oatmeal, or a small salad.

Protect Your Heart with Green tea + Lemon

In a study of more than 40,500 Japanese men and women, those who drank five or more cups of green tea every day had the lowest risk of dying of heart disease and stroke. This is very important to people with diabetes, who are at an increased risk of heart disease.

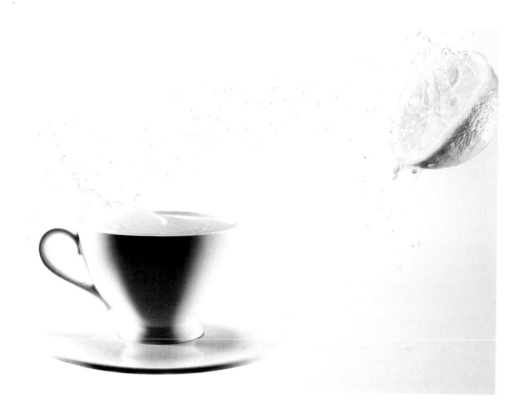

Researchers attribute the protective effect to catechins, powerful antioxidants. Trouble is, less than 20 percent of these relatively unstable compounds survive digestion. To get more out of every cup, squeeze in some lemon juice. The vitamin C in lemons helps your body absorb 13 times more catechins than it can obtain from plain tea alone, according to a Purdue University study.

Sip to your heart's content: With the catechin boost from vitamin C, you can help your heart by drinking just one or two cups daily. If lemons make you pucker, squeeze in some orange, lime, or grapefruit juice; they increase antioxidant absorption, too, though to a lesser extent.

Just skip the milk because it actually interferes with absorption. Stick to freshly brewed tea, hot or iced. The catechins in ready-to-drink bottles are ineffective.

Ward Off Heart Disease with the PLAC Test + hs-CRP Test

These tests measure Lp-PLA2 and CRP (C-reactive protein) levels, which are two important markers of the kind of inflammation caused by the accumulation of plaque in your arteries—a big predictor of heart disease. When doctors added the results of these screenings to their usual assessment of risk factors (blood pressure, cholesterol, etc.), they ended up reclassifying 39 percent of intermediate-risk patients—including 11 percent who were in need of more serious treatment—according to a new study published in the journal *Stroke*. Many of these patients may now be candidates for statins.

Get the tests if: You're middle-aged and your cholesterol is normal but you smoke, have gained weight, have a family history of heart disease, or have borderline hypertension, says Christie M. Ballantyne, MD, study coauthor and director of the Center for Cardiovascular Disease Prevention at Methodist DeBakey Heart & Vascular Center in Houston. If you do get put into a higher-risk category, statins aren't the only treatment. Both Lp-PLA2 and CRP levels respond well to diet and exercise.

Boost Brainpower with Exercise + Music

Twenty-one minutes of exercise is all it took to lift the moods of cardiac rehabilitation patients in an Ohio State University pilot study. But when participants listened to Antonio Vivaldi's *Four Seasons* on headphones, they performed significantly better on a verbal-fluency test afterward. Researchers believe that exercise boosts cognitive performance by stimulating the central nervous system, and the addition of music may help organize thoughts.

This is important for people with diabetes because diabetes increases the risk of getting Alzheimer's disease. It also might speed dementia once it strikes.

Move and groove: Though researchers haven't explored whether these findings can be generalized to apply to healthy adults, it can't hurt to exercise with your MP3 player. Stick to the same routine the study participants followed: Gradually increase the slope and speed on your treadmill every 10 minutes until you can speak only in short sentences. (Walk for a minimum of 21 minutes.) And listen to the music of your choice; any genre should work as effectively as classical.

Rev Immunity with Pot Roast + Carrots

Although experts don't think that diabetes decreases your immunity, anyone can benefit from a strong, healthy immune system, to better fight off bacteria and viruses.

This popular combination of comfort food makes you feel good for a reason. Carrots are chock-full of vitamin A, a retinol that plays a key role in preventing and fighting off infections. But without the zinc in the beef, your body wouldn't be able to use it. Vitamin A can travel through the blood only when it's bound to a protein.

"And zinc is required to make that retinol-binding protein," says Roberta Larson Duyff, RD, author of *American Dietetic Association Complete Food and Nutrition Guide*. "So if you don't have enough zinc, vitamin A is not going to move from the liver to the tissues, where it does its job."

Germ-fighting combos: Dark orange, yellow, red, and green fruits and vegetables are good sources of vitamin A. For a little lighter fare, pair them with zinc-rich proteins: Slice fresh mango into low-fat yogurt, eat a small sweet potato with your fish, or stuff your chicken with spinach, Florentine-style.

Flush Fat with a Burger + Frozen Yogurt

Nine in 10 people with diabetes are overweight. Yet losing weight and keeping it off can help you better manage your blood sugar. Eating a diet low in saturated fat can also help.

But the next time you *do* eat a food high in saturated fat, follow it with a low-fat, calcium-rich dessert. Calcium binds to fatty acids in the digestive tract, blocking their absorption. In one study, participants who ate 1,735 milligrams of calcium from low-fat dairy products (about as much as in five 8-ounce glasses of fat-free milk) blocked the equivalent of 85 calories a day.

Beef up calcium: Researchers haven't determined exactly how much calcium you should consume with each high-fat meal, says Cynthia Heiss, PhD, RD. "But by including a glass of fat-free or soy milk or a fortified juice with a fatty meal, you may get a boost if you're trying to lose weight," she says.

Save Your Eyesight with Salad + Avocado

Uncontrolled diabetes can harm your eyes, even causing blindness. Some of the diseases associated with diabetes are cataracts, glaucoma, and diabetic retinopathy.

Spinach may be good for your eyes, but avocado makes it even more effective. Researchers found that when adults ate a lettuce, spinach, and carrot salad with or without 3 tablespoons of avocado, the avocado eaters absorbed 8.3 times more alpha-carotene, 13.6 times more beta-carotene, and 4.3 times more lutein than the others. Researchers believe that the healthy fats in avocado increase the absorption of these fat-soluble carotenoids, which are associated with a decreased risk of macular degeneration and cataracts.

Go green: In the study, 3 tablespoons of avocado was nearly as effective as 6, so spare yourself the extra calories. Use a Hass avocado if possible because it has a higher monounsaturated fat content than other avocados. Or try swapping in another healthy fat source, such as safflower oil, nuts, or olives.

Build Muscle with Strength Training + Stretching

Exercise is key to managing diabetes. For people with diabetes, weight training helps increase glucose uptake by the muscles and helps the body store glucose. The stored form of glucose is called glycogen. Glycogen must be replenished after exercise, so anything that helps your body store glucose is a plus for people with diabetes. Weight training also increases your metabolism—even after you have finished with your workout. A faster metabolism helps you burn more calories, and it helps insulin work better, too.

Weight training builds strength by causing tiny tears in the muscle, which then quickly repairs itself, ending up bigger and stronger. Fast-track your strength gains by adding static stretching—in which you hold a stretch for 10 to 30 seconds—to your routine. Three studies led by *Prevention* advisor Wayne L. Westcott, PhD, fitness research director at Quincy College in Massachusetts, found that adults who stretched either between or

Health Update: Eggs

Eggs used to have a reputation as being a major culprit in heart disease risk, but current research says these claims are not all they're cracked up to be. Here's the truth behind three common myths.

Myth: Making eggs a regular part of your diet leads to heart disease.

Fact: Eating one egg per day barely affects your risk of heart disease, while factors such as physical inactivity and obesity increase it by as much as 40 percent, according to a recent study. The American Heart Association, however, does recommend keeping cholesterol consumption to less than 300 milligrams a day, so limit yourself to one whole egg daily. (The yolk contains approximately 213 milligrams.)

Myth: Egg yolks aren't healthy.

Fact: The yellow center is a rare source of vitamin D; just one has 20 IU as well as vitamin B_{12} and choline, among other nutrients. To keep cholesterol intake down, make your omelet with one whole egg and two whites, and watch cholesterol at the rest of your meals.

Myth: Brown-shelled eggs are nutritionally superior to white-shelled.

Fact: They're equal. White-shelled eggs are produced by hens with white feathers and white earlobes. Brown-shelled eggs are produced by hens with red feathers and red earlobes. Generally, red hens are slightly larger and need more food, so their eggs typically cost more.

immediately after strength-training exercises developed about 20 percent more strength than those who only lifted weights.

Lift and reach: Rest at least a minute between sets, and use that time to stretch the muscle you've just worked. For instance, if you just did leg extensions, stretch your quadriceps by pulling your right ankle toward your butt while standing on your left leg. Hold each stretch for 20 seconds.

Bolster Your Memory with Curcumin + Black Pepper

Diabetes has been implicated as a risk factor for eventually developing Alzheimer's, though experts don't quite yet understand the mysterious connection between these two conditions. But here's some good news: Some diabetes drugs appear to slow the cognitive decline associated with Alzheimer's disease.

Curcumin might be known for its anticancer properties, but this compound (found in the spice turmeric) is also making waves in Alzheimer's research. A recent study found that, compared with those who got a placebo, Alzheimer's patients who took 1 gram of curcumin either as a supplement or mixed with food reduced the buildup of plaque in their brains. However, curcumin tends to be poorly absorbed, so you'll need to mix it with black pepper to increase its absorption by up to 2,000 percent.

Spice up your palate: Turmeric has been used for centuries in Indian curries but may taste strong to an American palate. Start with ½ teaspoon daily, suggests Bharat B. Aggarwal, PhD, professor of cancer medicine at the University of Texas M. D. Anderson Cancer Center in Houston. Once you get used to the flavor, mix it with black pepper to make a great rub for fish or chicken.

Banish Breakouts with a Retinoid + Benzoyl Peroxide

When researchers combined adapalene, a retinoid that reduces inflammation, with benzoyl peroxide, which kills the bacteria that cause acne, study participants' acne improved, on average, by more than 50 percent in 12 weeks—about 15 percent better than with either ingredient alone.

"This new combination therapy targets three out of four causes of acne," says Diane M. Thiboutot, MD, professor of dermatology at the Penn State Milton S. Hershey Medical Center in Hershey.

The right regimen: Ask your doctor about Epiduo, the first FDA-approved acne product to combine adapalene (0.1%) and benzoyl peroxide (2.5%). Dr. Thiboutot recommends washing your face before bed with a gentle cleanser, waiting about 20 minutes, and then applying the gel, followed by a moisturizer. Epiduo can be drying, but any initial irritation should subside within 2 weeks. If you'd like to try an over-the-counter treatment, wash in the morning with a cleanser that contains benzoyl peroxide. We like PCA Skin pHaze 31 BPO 5% Cleanser (www.dermstore.com). At night, apply a serum containing retinol, such as Neova Retinol ME 0.15% (www.beautybridge.com). Retinols are milder versions of prescription retinoids.

Fight Fatigue with Eggs + Orange Juice

If you don't eat much meat, you might be feeling sluggish because you're not getting enough iron. Reason: Your body can readily absorb iron from meat (heme iron), but only 2 to 20 percent of the nonheme iron found in veggies, beans, and eggs makes it into your bloodstream. An effective booster: vitamin C.

"It's the most potent promoter of nonheme iron absorption," says Elaine Magee, MPH, RD, author of *Food Synergy*. Vitamin C keeps the iron up to six times more soluble—meaning your body can now use 100 percent of the nonheme iron you eat and stave off fatigue-causing anemia.

"C" that you get more iron: Wash down your morning omelet with a glass of C-rich orange juice. Or toss iron-rich tofu and C-dense broccoli into your salad. Keep the cooking to a minimum (or at low temperatures), and cut your produce into thick chunks. Vitamin C is easily destroyed by light, heat, and air.

Sidestep Skin Cancer with Caffeine + Cardio

Research shows that both caffeine and exercise have anticancer properties. Combined, they offer powerful protection against skin cancer. In research on animals exposed to UVB radiation, Rutgers University scientists learned that the pairing increased the animals' ability to destroy skin cancer cells by up to four times.

Allan H. Conney, PhD, director of the laboratory for cancer research at the Ernest Mario School of Pharmacy at Rutgers, suspects that caffeine inhibits ATR-1, a genetic pathway that prevents damaged cells from self-destructing. Both caffeine and exercise also decrease tissue fat, which research shows helps cells deconstruct.

Have a cup, then walk: Drink a strong cup of coffee an hour before exercise, recommends Monique Ryan, RD, author of *Sports Nutrition for Endurance Athletes*. (If your blood pressure is elevated, skip the caffeine.) Caffeine can also increase endurance and delay fatigue, helping you walk longer and stronger. Just don't forget the sunscreen.

CHAPTER

10

Consider These
SUPPLEMENTS

These natural remedies have ironclad scientific proof on their side. Here are two that everyone should consider, plus three others that benefit your bones, heart, and stomach—and even help control blood sugar.

Dietary supplements have officially gone mainstream. About two-thirds of Americans take them, and more than three-quarters of doctors recommend them to patients, according to recent surveys. Among the dizzying array of natural products found on pharmacy and health food store shelves, we've uncovered five truly outstanding complementary treatments in pill form that hold up to scientific scrutiny just as well as prescription drugs do.

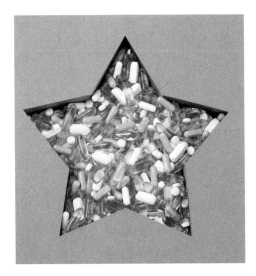

For Everyone: Fish Oil

The research: Talk about a heartfelt endorsement: "The only dietary supplement consistently shown in randomized clinical trials to work against cardiac death is fish oil," says Dariush Mozaffarian, MD, DrPH, assistant professor of cardiology and epidemiology at Harvard Medical School and the Harvard School of Public Health. Omega-3 fatty acids (commonly known as EPA and DHA)—found in salmon, tuna, and other fish—appear to fight cardiac death by stabilizing the heart's electrical system. Other benefits include lowering blood pressure and triglycerides, slowing arterial plaque buildup, and easing systemic inflammation. Fish oil was more successful than statins at preventing death in heart failure patients, according to a recent Italian study.

Bonus benefits: Research shows that omega-3s in fish oil may also help lower your risk of stroke and nonlethal heart attacks, relieve anxiety and depression, and reduce the risk of cognitive decline.

Try it: Because most Americans don't eat two servings of fish a week as suggested by the American Heart Association, many experts recommend taking a daily supplement containing 1,000 milligrams of EPA and DHA combined (even if you are a fan of fish).

"The main side effect is fishy burps, but storing softgels in the freezer and taking them with food can help," Dr. Mozaffarian advises. Nearly all commercial fish oil brands are reliably safe, but check labels for the EPA and DHA amounts per serving.

For Everyone: Vitamin D

The research: It's suddenly one of the most popular vitamins on the planet, and for good reason: Up to 53 percent of us may not get enough vitamin D from sources such as direct sunlight and food (fish and fortified dairy, for example), reports the National Institutes of Health, and the current guideline of 400 IU daily has recently been dismissed by experts as insufficient.

That's because this nutrient has wide-ranging health impacts: More than 1,000 human and lab studies indicate that vitamin D not only augments calcium absorption but also may ward off breast, colorectal, ovarian, and other cancers. And getting too little vitamin D could cause premature death from heart disease, according to a recent study.

"Vitamin D has really gotten the attention of the medical community," says Michael F. Holick, MD, PhD, director of the Bone Health Care Clinic at Boston University School of Medicine.

Bonus benefits: Getting more vitamin D may also lower your risk of developing autoimmune diseases such as type 1 diabetes, multiple sclerosis, and rheumatoid arthritis, studies have found. And not getting enough has been linked to bone, joint, and muscle pain; fibromyalgia; and osteoarthritis.

Try it: Take vitamin D as a supplement because food and sun are rarely sufficient, particularly if you live in northern states that get little daily solar radiation during the winter.

"If you take 1,000 IU a day and get 5 to 10 minutes of unblocked sun a few times a week, you're almost guaranteed to get enough," says Dr. Holick.

Supermarket and pharmacy brands are considered safe and effective and cost pennies per pill.

For People with High Cholesterol: Reducol

The research: Plant sterol and stanol compounds in a healthy diet can lower LDL (bad) cholesterol by as much as 20 percent—comparable to the effects of statin drugs. But the small amounts in fruits, vegetables, nuts, and seeds aren't always enough to provide the 2 grams daily of sterols and stanols that the American Heart Association suggests for people with high cholesterol, which can increase the risk of heart disease. Foods containing manufactured sterol-and-stanol blends such as Reducol can help.

In one study, Reducol added to margarine lowered LDL cholesterol by 15 percent. Fat in foods helps absorption of sterols and stanols, but Reducol pills may also help (e.g., Nature Made CholestOff and Twinlab Cholesterol Success, both in 900-milligram doses).

"The pills aren't as effective as food, but they can still lower LDL cholesterol by up to 10 percent," says Peter J. H. Jones,

PhD, director of the Richardson Centre for Functional Foods and Nutraceuticals at Canada's University of Manitoba.

Bonus benefits: Initial evidence suggests that sterols and stanols might reduce the risk of breast, colon, and stomach cancers. For now, though, ask your doctor before taking Reducol for any reason other than your cholesterol.

Try it: "I recommend 900 milligrams three times per day for high cholesterol, and then reduce the dose to 450 milligrams three times per day if LDL numbers are coming down," says New York physician Fred Pescatore, MD, author of *The Hamptons Diet*. Dr. Pescatore puts nearly all of his patients on Reducol, even as a preventive measure (900 milligrams once per day in that case). Some products, such as Country Life TLC (aka Cardia-

Beat), now combine sterols and omega-3s in a single pill.

For People with Tummy Trouble: Culturelle

The research: Culturelle is one of the most researched probiotics on the planet. The only US dietary supplement containing the active culture lactobacillus GG (LGG), it acts directly on the immune system and helps ward off viral illness; replaces good bacteria killed in the intestines during antibiotic therapy; and keeps harmful bacteria, fungi, parasites, and other infectious microorganisms in check. (It eliminated up to 47 percent of traveler's diarrhea in two studies.) Culturelle survives unusually well in stomach acid to colonize the intestine and contains 10 billion live cells per

FOUR SUSPECT SUPPLEMENTS

Ask your doctor before taking any of these in pill form. You're probably already getting what you need from a healthy diet and a multivitamin.

Folic acid: It can help prevent birth defects, but a 2007 study found that 1 milligram daily (that's more than twice the recommended levels) via supplements may raise colon cancer risk. Done having kids? Get your 400 micrograms daily from most grains and cereals.

Vitamin E: A 2008 study found that taking supplements of vitamin E might increase the risk of lung cancer, especially among smokers. Also, more than a dozen common prescription meds can interact with high doses of E.

Selenium: Consuming more than 400 micrograms a day raises the risk of premature death, according to a Johns Hopkins University study; many selenium pills contain half this amount. Another study linked selenium to the development of type 2 diabetes after 7 years of supplementation.

Beta-carotene: Several studies indicate that taking beta-carotene supplements may increase the risk of cancer or heart disease.

dose—10 times more than most yogurts.

"That's important because probiotics can't help keep your gut healthy if they don't last, and few do as well as LGG," says Jon Vanderhoof, MD, a professor emeritus at the University of Nebraska College of Medicine in Omaha.

In a recent Australian trial, people who ate yogurt containing LGG cleared antibiotic-resistant bacteria from the gut in 4 weeks, while those eating yogurt without it did not.

Although people with diabetes don't necessarily have decreased immunity, anyone would be happy to have a better immune system and fight off infections.

Bonus benefits: Studies suggest that LGG might also ease irritable bowel syndrome.

Try it: Follow Culturelle's dose instruction of one capsule per day. Refrigerating the supplement isn't required, though doing so may increase its shelf life. As intestinal flora begins to change, side effects such as bloating and gas usually disappear in a few days.

For People with Joint Pain: Pycnogenol

The research: This extract from French maritime pine bark is cited in more than 200 studies and continues to impress researchers. In two recent trials, osteoar-

thritis patients who took Pycnogenol for 3 months reduced their pain and stiffness by 35 to 55 percent and needed fewer drugs such as NSAIDs or COX-2 inhibitors. Pycnogenol's efficacy is probably due to its having both antioxidant and anti-inflammatory properties.

"Pycnogenol's compounds are especially potent, yet there aren't really side effects," says Sherma Zibadi, MD, a graduate research associate who studied the extract at the University of Arizona's College of Public Health in Tucson.

If you have diabetes, you're at increased risk of various bone and joint disorders. Factors such as nerve damage (diabetic neuropathy), arterial disease, and obesity all may contribute to these problems. But often the cause isn't clear.

Bonus benefits: Pycnogenol wards off heart disease by lowering LDL and raising HDL (good) cholesterol, reducing blood pressure and risk of clotting, and controlling blood sugar in people with type 2 diabetes. It also reduced menstrual aches in one study, cutting days spent on pain meds in half. A new study shows that it may even help fend off jet lag.

Try it: Take a 50-milligram tablet two or three times daily with meals. Ask your doctor before you start, especially if you're on hypertension meds—and don't take more than 200 milligrams a day, Dr. Zibaldi says.

PART

3

LOSE

Losing weight might be your best

WEIGHT

first step in managing diabetes.

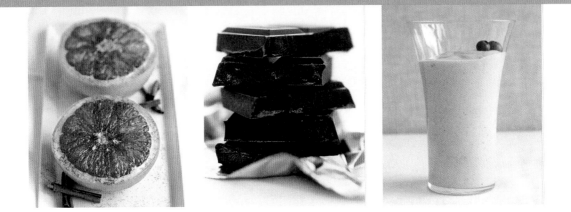

WEIGHT LOSS
Medical Breakthroughs

If you're overweight and have diabetes, losing weight can help you control your blood sugar, possibly even get off medications. And it might not even take a dramatic weight loss. **Experts say that if people who have diabetes lose 5 to 10 percent of their weight, they will significantly reduce their blood sugar.**

CHECK YOUR WEIGHT

A normal BMI (body mass index) doesn't necessarily mean a slim chance of developing diabetes or heart disease. In a recent study published in the *Archives of Internal Medicine,* one-quarter of normal-weight adults had a trio of symptoms—high blood pressure, triglycerides, and blood glucose—that put them at risk of cardiovascular and metabolic disease.

Talk with your doctor about preventing heart disease and diabetes, particularly if you have any of these risk factors: a family history of either disease; an apple-shaped body; or African American, Native American, or Latino ethnicity. She may recommend staying active, not smoking, and consuming more heart-healthy foods.

BEWARE DOCTOR BIAS

Physicians were 14 percent less likely to respect patients for every 10 points higher their BMI was, found a recent study from Johns Hopkins University School of Medicine.

"Other data show that doctors who don't respect patients share less medical information with them, and these patients play a smaller role in making decisions about their health," says study author Mary Margaret Huizinga, MD, MPH. If you don't feel comfortable with your doc, shop around for someone with whom you have a better rapport.

DODGE DIET BUSTERS

"Lite" meals at restaurants might actually be bursting with diet-busting calories. Many contain an average of 18 percent more than menus claim, report Tufts University researchers who analyzed the calorie content of 29 dishes promoted as "healthy" on national sit-down and fast-food menus. If you eat out three times a week, the following could pack on a 4-pound weight gain in a year.

Larger portions. Watch for thicker cuts of meat and extra veggies—even the calories in healthy foods can add up.

DODGE 'EM. If your serving looks oversize, save half the meal before you start or leave a few bites on your plate.

Taste enhancers. Hoping to boost flavor, chefs may add more oil, butter, cream, or sugar than the recipe calls for.

DODGE 'EM. Ask for sauces and dressings on the side, and use them sparingly.

Free sides. Oily french fries and mayo-packed pasta salads often contain more calories than the dish you ordered.

DODGE 'EM. Avoid any extras listed separately on the menu.

SLIM DOWN LIKE CLOCKWORK

The key to maintaining a healthy weight is not just what you eat but when you eat it. People who consistently eat at the same times each day—and don't skip meals—are less likely to develop a large waistline or insulin resistance (factors in developing type 2 diabetes), according to a study of 3,607 women and men by the Karolinska Institute in Sweden. Conversely, people who skip meals or eat at odd hours have a higher risk of metabolic disease.

REV UP YOUR METABOLISM

Consider the following metabolism boosters.

Citrus: Researchers believe that the flavonoid naringenin, which is abundant in citrus fruits such as oranges and grapefruit, might promote weight loss, according to a new animal study from the University of Western Ontario. Supplementing a high-fat diet with naringenin lowered elevated blood sugar and high cholesterol, thwarted the onset of insulin resistance, and prevented obesity. The researchers also found that adding large amounts of this flavonoid to the diet caused the liver to burn excess fat rather than store it.

Vinegar: The primary substance that gives ordinary vinegar its sour taste and strong odor may fight fat, suggests new research presented at a recent meeting of the Japanese Society of Nutrition and Food Science. In a study of 175 overweight Japanese men and women, those who consumed a drink containing either 1 or 2 tablespoons of apple cider vinegar daily for 12 weeks had significantly lower body weight, BMI, visceral fat, and waist circumference than the control group that didn't consume any vinegar. Researchers credit vinegar's acetic acid, which may

switch on genes that pump out proteins that break down fat.

QUELL CRAVINGS ALL DAY

Try these smart meal-by-meal strategies to sidestep mindless snacking.

At breakfast: Scramble some eggs and chase them with milk. Researchers at the University of Connecticut found that adults who ate eggs rather than a bagel in the morning consumed fewer calories all day and felt satisfied longer. And people who downed $2^1/_2$ cups of fat-free milk with their breakfast reported reduced appetite and decreased calorie intake at lunch, according to a study in the *American Journal of Clinical Nutrition.*

At lunch: Forgo rice in your burrito or trade chips for fruit to reduce your intake of refined carbohydrates. A small daily reduction in the amount of carb calories—from 55 to 43 percent—increases the sense of fullness, report researchers from the University of Alabama at Birmingham.

At snack time: Eat some dark chocolate. It may help you feel full, according to a new study from Denmark. Researchers gave 16 participants 100 grams of either dark or milk chocolate and 2 hours later offered them pizza. Those who consumed the dark chocolate ate 15 percent less calories than those who had milk chocolate, and they were less interested in fatty, salty, and sugary foods. Try a chocolate with 70 percent or more cocoa. Two tablespoons of dark chocolate chips alongside

The average number of pounds people lost after practicing yoga for 8 weeks:

6

fresh berries as a midafternoon snack should give you some of the benefits without breaking your calorie budget.

At dinner: Add olive oil and avocado. These healthy fats can boost satiety. It's a misconception that a low-fat supper is good for your waistline. Consuming fatty foods—particularly mono- and polyunsaturated fats—activates a compound in the small intestine that halts hunger, suggests University of California, Irvine, research. So don't be afraid to spritz your steamed veggies with olive oil.

▦ TRY YOGA

People who practice yoga are more likely to eat mindfully—noshing only when physically hungry and stopping when full, suggests a study from the Fred Hutchinson Cancer Research Center. This may be why they also weigh about 15 pounds less than people who don't do the Downward-Facing Dog.

Researchers believe that yoga cultivates an awareness of emotional and physical sensations that makes you more conscious of your food choices. Get started at www.prevention.com/hungeryoga.

▦ USE YOUR BRAIN

Attention, emotional eaters: Cultivating an optimistic outlook can keep your diet on track, report researchers at the universities of Chicago and Michigan.

In a recent study, participants who were happy but believed that their good moods would be short-lived were more likely to choose chocolate instead of an apple. Similarly, unhappy participants tended to opt for the caloric snack when they expected their sadness to persist. Don't let emotions dictate your diet: If you're feeling upbeat, focus on why the good feeling will last; if you're unhappy, think of reasons the sadness will pass.

▦ SUBSTITUTE MUSHROOMS FOR MEAT

Here's an easy swap to drastically cut calories: Trade the beef in your recipes for mushrooms. Research from Johns Hopkins University showed that when adults ate a mushroom-based version of four beef dishes such as lasagna and chili, they were not only just as full but also ate around 420 fewer calories and 30 fewer grams of fat. Substituting 1 cup of mushrooms for 3 ounces of 85 percent lean ground meat twice a week could add up to a 6-pound weight loss over 1 year.

▦ BOOST YOUR CALCIUM

Boosting your calcium intake may help curb your appetite and make slimming down easier, suggests research in the *British Journal of Nutrition*. When calcium-deficient women took a supplement, they lost four times more weight than those who didn't take the extra calcium. Researchers believe that the brain compensates for a calcium shortage by initiating hunger to encourage eating foods that are rich in the mineral. Because most women fall short on calcium, aim to consume fat-free or low-fat

The number of calories in 1 cup of grilled sliced portobello mushrooms:

42

yogurt and milk, beans, and dark leafy greens throughout the day, or talk with your doctor about supplements.

▒ AVOID BRAIN BINGE

Overeating at work? There may be a reason: Intellectual activities make people munch more. Students who performed a series of memory, attention, and vigilance tests ate 253 more calories than students who relaxed for the same amount of time, found researchers at Laval University in Quebec.

The reason? Intellectual work causes larger fluctuations in blood sugar levels, and that can stir up the urge to nibble. To reduce your drive to eat when you're in thinking mode, try keeping a water bottle or healthy snack nearby to help keep blood sugar steady while you work.

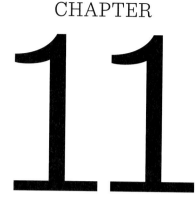
Slim Down to Say "GOOD-BYE, DIABETES"

What's weight got to do with it? A lot, it turns out!

D iabetes and obesity are intertwined like the pieces of a buttery soft pretzel. People with diabetes are more likely to be overweight, and having diabetes makes it harder to lose weight.

At its core, diabetes is about blood sugar—or, more precisely, badly behaved blood sugar, the kind that likes to soar high and then plunge low, like an amusement park roller coaster. Except this ride is no fun because it leaves you tired and mentally fuzzy and maybe just a little cranky. It's also playing games with your weight.

You see, high blood sugar is a hallmark of insulin resistance, in which insulin can't do its job of escorting blood sugar into cells. Insulin resistance is a common precursor to diabetes. It also can make weight loss that much harder.

Getting rid of those extra pounds helps your body's cells respond to insulin more effectively. Insulin, you'll remember, is the hormone that escorts glucose—blood sugar—out of your bloodstream and into cells, where it's turned into energy.

When insulin does its job, it keeps a tight rein on blood sugar, which means fewer peaks and valleys. Instead, your blood sugar stays on an even keel—and pounds melt away faster and easier.

The Belly Fat-Blood Sugar Connection

Turns out that not all fat is created equal. One type—visceral fat—is particularly dangerous. Visceral fat doesn't jiggle when you dance. It won't spill over the waistband of your skinny jeans. And it's not the stuff of love handles, little belly pooches, muffin tops, or "pinching an inch" at your waistline.

This most dangerous fat in your body lies deep within your abdomen, beneath your skin, behind puffy subcutaneous fat (the fat you can notice on your waist, hips, thighs, etc.), and under your abdominal muscles. Doctors catch glimpses of it only during major surgical procedures. Researchers who use high-tech magnetic resonance imaging (MRI) machines and computed tomography (CT) scanning equipment to measure visceral fat say that everyone has a little bit—it protects organs and may even play a role in immunity. However, if you're overweight, you might have several pounds of it.

Visceral fat is not benign. The *v* in visceral fat truly stands for *vicious*. Medical experts now say this deep belly fat is strongly associated with diabetes and prediabetes, as well as with metabolic syndrome, which is a common and often overlooked condition that leads to both. It also contributes to high blood pressure, heart disease, strokes, and even dementia and some forms of cancer.

It's no wonder, then, that when it comes to health, researchers say we should worry about hidden visceral fat, not the subcutaneous fat padding your waist, hips, thighs, arms, and butt. Of course, if you're hoping to fit back into your skinny jeans, you're going to worry about both.

Location, Location, Location

Why is visceral fat so deadly? In part because it occupies some prime real estate within your abdomen.

It's no coincidence that the word *visceral* comes from *viscera,* which is the Latin word for "internal organs." Visceral fat cozies right up against the organs that keep you alive and well—and that keep your blood sugar on an even keel. Connected by tiny blood vessels to your portal vein—the so-called super highway that delivers blood to your heart, liver, and other internal organs—visceral fat affects the important functions of these organs in ways that subcutaneous fat does not.

We're not talking about a little dab of fat. When researchers in Hong Kong measured visceral fat with MRI machines, they discovered layers $^1/_2$ to 1 inch thick in people who were about 5 to 20 pounds overweight. Less is better; researchers have found that the risk of metabolic syndrome begins to rise when visceral fat is just $^4/_{10}$ inch thick. Your age, gender, and genes all play roles in how much fat you store deep in your abdomen, but body weight plays a big role. The more you weigh, the more visceral fat you're likely to have.

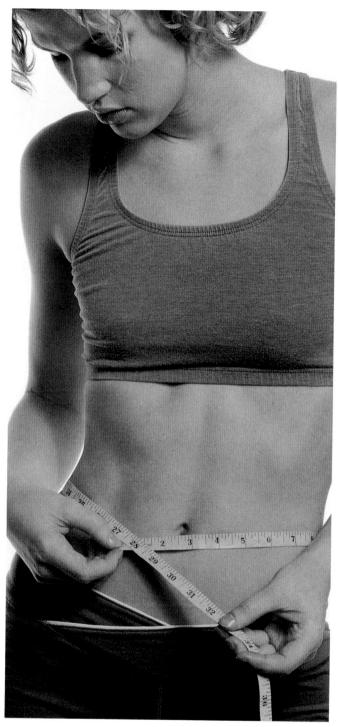

The Toxic Chemical Factory in Your Torso

The second reason visceral fat is so dangerous is that it's active fat. Scientists used to think that the human body's 40 billion to 120 billion fat cells were like the plastic containers in your refrigerator, just holding extra calories until needed.

Today we know that fat is more like the leaky faucet on your kitchen sink; it drips constantly. Sometimes the "drip" benefits our health: A recent announcement from Harvard Medical School stated that subcutaneous fat—such as hip fat, thigh fat, butt fat, and the fat just below the skin on your belly—might produce substances that protect against diabetes.

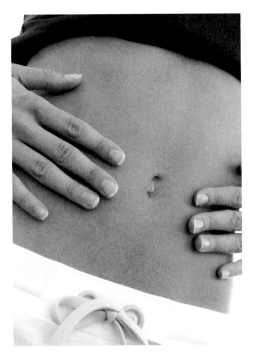

But visceral fat's drip also churns out dozens of chemicals and hormones that interfere with the healthy functioning of your liver, heart, and pancreas, as well as your blood vessels, muscle cells, and even brain. They also affect the tissue in a woman's breasts and in a man's prostate gland.

Insulin, Blood Sugar, and Belly Fat

What does all this mean for you? To understand deep belly fat's implications for diabetes, you must understand how your body handles blood sugar when everything's operating properly.

When you eat a meal, such as a quick lunch consisting of a tuna fish sandwich, an apple, a cookie, and a glass of milk, your digestive system converts the carbohydrates from the bread, the fruit, the cookie, and even the milk into blood sugar. This is your body's primary source of fuel.

Getting that fuel into cells is insulin's job. Normally your pancreas—which is a cone-shaped, spongy, 6-inch-long organ located just behind your liver—produces this hormone and releases a squirt when blood sugar levels begin to rise after you eat. Insulin tells cells to open up and let the sugar in. And normally your cells obey.

But if your body stops obeying insulin's commands, you begin developing insulin resistance. That means your cells may not respond readily to the insulin you take, requiring you to use more and making daily blood sugar control more challenging.

It makes sense, then, that an eating or exercise plan that fights deep visceral fat could help you fight insulin resistance and remain sensitive to the insulin you use to keep your blood sugar in control.

The good news: Losing even a little of this dangerous belly fat can make your blood sugar easier to control. In one study of 114 people with type 2 diabetes who used oral medications to control their blood sugar, those who lost just 15 percent of their weight needed less medication because their cells became three times more sensitive to insulin.

Belly Fat and Other Big Health Risks

Blood sugar problems are just part of the story. The following serious health problems have also been associated with higher levels of visceral fat.

Yes, There Is Good Body Fat

Your body needs a little padding to function. Without it you'd freeze in a winter wind, have trouble healing from the smallest cut or scrape, run out of energy between meals, and run the risk of damaging your internal organs just by bumping into a kitchen counter. An estimated 2 to 5 percent of a man's body weight comes from "essential" fat; for women, it's 10 to 15 percent. Body fat's metabolic benefits include the following:

- Providing energy
- Maintaining proper hormone levels
- Regulating body temperature
- Protecting vital organs
- Aiding fertility
- Stimulating bone growth
- Boosting immunity and healing
- Releasing hormones that regulate appetite

Plus, Harvard Medical School researchers, in a study published in the journal *Cell Metabolism*, recently found that a mysterious factor in the fat just below the skin (a type of fat called subcutaneous fat) might protect against diabetes.

FAT IS NOT YOUR FATE

Research suggests that, by and large, our genes determine our weight range. But lifestyle—what we eat, how much we move—determines where we fall within that range.

Translation: You're not destined to be overweight, even if all your relatives happen to be. In general, lifestyle trumps genetics. For proof, we need look no further than the Pima Indians of Arizona and Mexico.

Extensive studies of this population provide a great example of the interplay between genetics and lifestyle. Both Arizonan and Mexican Pimas are genetically predisposed to type 2 diabetes. Researchers have learned, for example, that Pimas carry a gene called FABP2 that might play a role in insulin resistance. Other studies have shown that another gene linked to type 2 diabetes and insulin resistance is more common in Pimas than in whites.

But what a difference a Western lifestyle makes. Arizonan Pimas have the highest prevalence of type 2 diabetes on Earth. Fully half of those between ages 30 and 64 have diabetes, and 95 percent of those with diabetes are overweight.

However, in a landmark 2006 study, researchers at the University of Wisconsin–Milwaukee discovered that Mexican Pimas have dramatically lower rates of diabetes and obesity. These two groups share a common genetic background, but their eating habits and levels of physical activity are strikingly different.

As a result, the obesity rate among Arizonan Pima men is 10 times higher than that of their Mexican counterparts. In fact, the obesity and diabetes rates among Mexican Pimas are comparable to the rates among other Mexicans with similar lifestyles. That's because Mexican Pimas eat about the same number of calories and grams of fiber as other Mexicans, and they tend to lead very active lifestyles. Arizonan Pimas, on the other hand, have adopted the lifestyle habits of most Americans—heavy on calorie-laden foods, light on exercise.

So don't blame your genes for putting you at risk of overweight and diabetes. Outsmart them with a healthy lifestyle!

Heart attack and stroke: If you have diabetes, prediabetes, or metabolic syndrome, the health of your heart should be one of your top priorities. Blood sugar and insulin problems go hand in hand with cardiovascular problems—and visceral fat is involved. A wide waist (more than 35 inches for women)—an indicator of visceral fat deep inside your torso—tripled the risk of fatal heart disease in a Harvard Medical School study of 44,636 women. The same connection has been found in men. Visceral fat threatens your cardiovascular system in several ways. Researchers have found that it quadruples your risk of high blood pressure and raises your risk of high levels of "lousy" LDL and low levels of "helpful" HDL cholesterol by 30 to 100 percent.

Cancer: Visceral fat increases risk of

cancers of the breast, prostate, and colon. The connection? Experts suspect it's excess insulin, which acts like a growth factor and encourages cells to grow and divide. A big waistline also makes it more likely that you would not survive cancer treatment, Harvard researchers have found.

Dementia: Visceral fat also increases your odds for developing dementia. When researchers at the Kaiser Permanente Division of Research in Oakland, California, tracked more than 6,000 people, they found that those with big bellies were 65 percent more likely to develop fuzzy thinking and memory lapses later in life than those with the slimmest midlines. The link in this case? The researchers suspect it may be inflammation.

Exercise, Belly Fat, and Blood Sugar

Have you moved around much today? If you haven't weeded the garden, walked the dog, gone to the gym, or gotten some other type of physical activity, put this book down immediately and treat yourself to a 5-minute stroll.

Back already? You've just taken an important step in vanquishing visceral fat. The fact is, leading a sedentary life is a big contributor to the worldwide expansion of waistlines. We know you're busy, and we know it's tough to find a half hour for exercise. But the fact is, any kind of activity helps fight this fat, even if you're fitting in a couple of 10-minute walks per day, making a point of finding time to dance along to the radio, or spending a sweaty 20 minutes planting green beans in your vegetable garden.

While everyone deserves time to unwind in front of the TV, you need to balance screen time with activity: Harvard School of Public Health researchers have found that every 2 hours a day in front of the tube boosts risk of insulin resistance by 23 percent! (Of course, exercising while you watch DVDs, as in the workouts in Chapter 19, solves that problem neatly!)

The Number You Must Know

Wondering whether there's bad fat lurking in your midsection? Someday soon, your doctor may be able to scan your torso or even check your blood to find out. Researchers at Beth Israel Deaconess Medical Center have discovered elevated levels of a telltale protein called RBP4 in people with excess visceral fat, a finding

Quick Tip

To curb soda cravings, try a seltzer-juice combo with no added sugar. Or keep a pitcher of water in the fridge. Add slices of orange, lemon, lime, or cucumber to give it kick.

	Healthy Range	At Risk of Diabetes and Heart Disease	High Risk
Men	Below 37 in	37–39 in	40 in and above
Women	Below 32 in	32–34 in	35 in and above
Asian men	Below 30 in	30–35 in	35½ in and above
Asian women	Below 28 in	28–31 in	31½ in and above

Note: Experts recommend smaller waist sizes for people of Asian descent because of a higher genetic risk for diabetes and cardiovascular disease. Studies show that this risk rises for Asians even at lower body weights and smaller waist sizes because of an inherited pattern of abdominal fat storage.

that could lead to a "belly fat test" someday. For now we've got a simpler method. Put down this book for a moment and go grab a soft, flexible tape measure, the kind used for sewing.

Your waist size is easy to measure; plus, studies show that it's a very accurate picture of your visceral fat status. When Brazilian researchers used CT scanners to measure visceral fat in 100 women and then checked their weight, waist size, and skinfold thickness with calipers (like those used in many gyms to check body fat), they discovered that waist size really did accurately reflect the amount of visceral fat inside a woman's torso.

The first thing to remember about checking your visceral fat status is that it's not the same as measuring to see if you're ready for a bathing suit or to check what size pants to buy. Honesty and accuracy really count—no cinching, sucking in your breath, or knocking off a half inch because you're feeling a little bloated! And you won't necessarily measure your

waist at its narrowest point or use your belly button as a landmark for lining up the tape.

For the most accurate belly fat reading, the National Institutes of Health recommends using the tops of your hip bones instead. This ensures that you'll measure across the section of your abdomen that hides significant amounts of visceral fat.

Here's what to do.

1. Measure on bare skin. Strip to your birthday suit, or take off your shirt and unfasten your pants. Push your pants and underwear down past your hips. (Squeezing tight pants down onto your hips while you measure isn't a good idea—you could get a "muffin top" bulge that makes your waist seem bigger than it really is!)

2. Stand in front of a mirror with your feet shoulder-width apart. Be sure you can see your waist and hips in the mirror.

3. Use your hands to find the uppermost points on your hip bones. Wrap the measuring tape around your middle so that the bottom edge rests just above

these bones. Pull the tape in snug and straight, not twisted or tight.

4. Relax and take two or three normal breaths. Take your measurement at the end of the third exhalation.

5. Write the number here: _____ inches (to the nearest ¼ inch).

6. Recheck around once a month.

Check our chart to see how your waist rates.

And Now for the Good News

Visceral fat, it turns out, is easier to lose than the fat on our hips, thighs, and bottoms. Research shows that just a little bit of weight loss adds up to big losses of deep abdominal fat—and big health benefits, including better insulin sensitivity, less need for diabetes medications, lower blood pressure, healthy cholesterol levels, and a lower risk of developing diabetes.

In study after study, women and men who've taken smart, belly fat–banishing steps saw dramatic reductions in their waist sizes and even bigger drops in the amount of visceral fat lurking below their waistbands. Losing belly fat really does improve your health. Here's how.

Less insulin resistance: In a study from Finland, losing visceral fat improved insulin sensitivity by 17 percent. A change like that could mean you'd need a lower dose of blood sugar–lowering medication

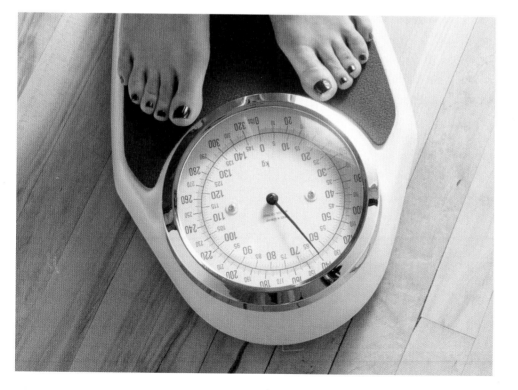

if you have diabetes now, or you would have a significantly lower risk of ever developing diabetes if you don't.

Reduced risk of progressing from prediabetes to diabetes: Losing abdominal fat was the secret to the success of the landmark Diabetes Prevention Program study, which followed 3,234 people with prediabetes. Researchers recently found that study participants who made healthy lifestyle changes—they ate less saturated fat and more fiber, cut calories, and exercised—reduced their visceral fat by 18 to 22 percent and cut their risk of developing full-blown diabetes by 58 percent.

Protection from heart attacks and strokes: In a Canadian study, women who lost visceral fat also saw two important signs of cardiovascular health improve: Levels of helpful HDLs rose by 50 to 65 percent, and blood pressure fell by 5 to 11 percent.

Dropping visceral fat pampers your heart in other ways, too. In an Australian study of 18 people—9 with diabetes and 9 with normal blood sugar—those who lost weight and trimmed their waistlines saw levels of heart-threatening triglycerides fall by about 18 percent.

Less inflammation: Chronic, low-level inflammation is a culprit behind major health conditions ranging from diabetes and heart attacks to strokes and cancer. Losing belly fat reduces signs of inflammation significantly, studies show.

In one from the University of Vermont, women who lost visceral fat saw levels of C-reactive protein (CRP)—an important marker of chronic, low-level inflammation—fall by 33 percent. And it doesn't take much weight loss or belly fat loss to get these results. In the Diabetes Prevention Program, women and men who lost just 7 percent of their body weight—that's a little more than 12 pounds if you now weigh 175—saw CRP levels drop by 29 to 33 percent.

Get Your Slimmest
BODY!

Yes, you can **smooth cellulite, drop 10 pounds, and firm up in just 8 weeks.** Our readers tested this groundbreaking plan.

Get ready for a total-body transformation!

With this shaping plan, you can shrink a whole size (or two!), tone trouble spots, and smooth out annoying dimples so you'll look and feel great when you slip on your shortest shorts!

At the heart of the plan is a science-backed strength-and-cardio routine designed to target the areas you want to firm up the most: your legs, butt, and belly. Because these are some of your biggest muscles, you'll also burn more calories to lose weight all over. *Prevention* advisor Wayne Westcott, PhD, fitness research director at Quincy College in Massachusetts, has found that this type of below-the-belt training, especially when combined with cardio and a healthy diet (which you'll find here, too), also minimizes cellulite in just 2 months. In one study of 115 women, he reported a reduction in cellulite in all the women, and ultrasound measurements revealed a higher proportion of muscle to fat in their legs. Even better, combining strength training and cardio into one workout can help exercisers curb their appetites to the tune of 500 fewer calories a day.

To guarantee that it works, we had readers give it a try.

"I lost 10 pounds and lots of tummy fat," says Kathryn Townsend, 37, of Kempton, Pennsylvania. "I went down two sizes, and my friends tell me I look younger." Sounds like the perfect way to get in shape.

Program at a Glance

THE WORKOUT
What you'll need: A stability ball, mat, and step

3 nonconsecutive days a week: Do the two-part Summer-Body Workout (30 to 45 minutes total).

4 days a week: Do at least 30 minutes of moderate-intensity activity such as yoga, hiking, dancing, or playing volleyball or other fun sports.

THE DIET
Follow our satisfying 1,800-calorie Summer-Body Diet on page 112.

THE EXPERTS
Craig Ballantyne, CSCS, author of *Turbulence Training*, who has helped thousands of women get beach ready, designed this workout.

Dermatologist David E. Bank, MD, author of *Beautiful Skin*, helps the Federal Trade Commission review cellulite products and treatments; he assessed our test panel.

SUMMER-BODY WORKOUT Part 1: Fast Firming

This routine minimizes rest time and maximizes calorie burn and toning. Do the six moves that follow in pairs (or supersets) without a break between exercises. Then rest 1 minute before performing the next pair. Start with 1 set of the recommended reps for each superset, adding a set each week until you're up to 3 sets, with a 1-minute break between sets if needed. Warm up with light activity such as marching in place for 5 minutes.

Superset 1

Hands-Up Squat

15 reps

> (A) Stand with your feet more than shoulder-width apart and your fingers laced behind your head, keeping your elbows back.

> (B) Bend at your hips and knees and lower until your thighs are almost parallel to the ground. Press back to standing.
> (C) Challenge yourself: From the down position, explode upward, jumping a few inches off the ground, landing softly with your knees slightly bent.

A

B

C

Superset 1

Single-Leg Bridge

12 reps per side

> Lie with your knees bent, feet flat, arms at your sides. (A) Extend your right leg, keeping your knees aligned. (B) Tighten your abs, contract your left glute, and lift your hips off the ground so that your body forms a straight line from knees to shoulders. Slowly lower your hips without touching the ground.

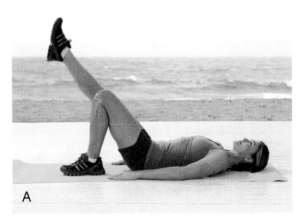

A

Quick Tip

Two low-cost ways to minimize cellulite, from Miami Beach–based dermatologist Leslie Baumann, MD: Professional deep-tissue massage (that uses harder pressure) and inverted yoga poses like shoulder stands (see www. prevention.com/inverted) help improve lymph flow, which can lessen the appearance of cellulite.

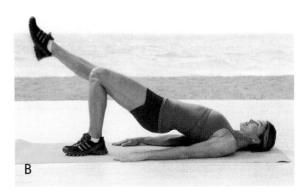

B

Step-Up

15 reps per side

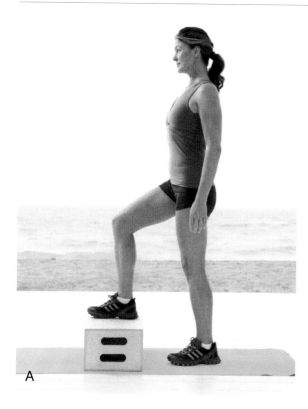

A

> ❯ (A) Face a bench or high step (about 12 inches) with your right foot on top, knee directly over ankle, and foot flat. (B) Press into your right foot and lift your body onto the bench, tapping it with your left toes. Keep your abs tight and don't lean forward. Slowly lower to the starting position.

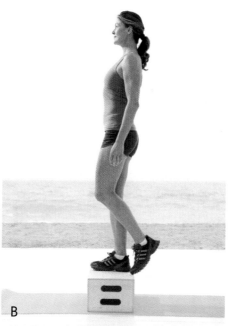

B

Superset 2

Stability Ball Leg Curl

12 reps

> Lie with your heels on a stability ball. (A)
  Contract your abs and glutes and lift your
  hips off the ground so that your body
  forms a straight line. (B) Bend your knees
  and roll the ball toward your hips. Pause,
  then extend your legs, keeping your hips
  lifted the entire time.

> **Challenge yourself:** Do single-leg curls,
  keeping your opposite leg raised in the air.

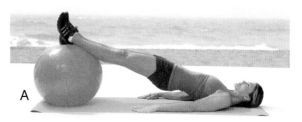

A

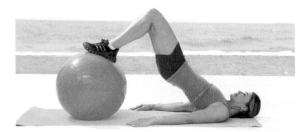

B

Split Squat

8 reps per side

> (A) Stand 2 to 3 feet in front of a bench with the top of your left foot on the bench. (B) Keeping your abs tight, bend your right leg and lower it until your front thigh is parallel to the ground. Keep your front knee behind your toes and don't lean forward. Press back to standing.

Quick Tip

Next to a pair of Bermuda shorts, the best way to hide cellulite is with self-tanner. A darker skin tone will make shadows from uneven skin less noticeable, giving you a smooth look.

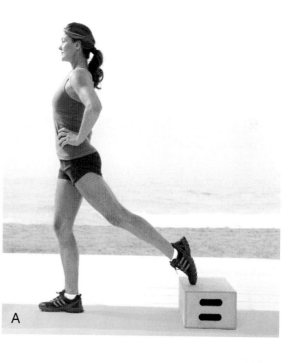

A

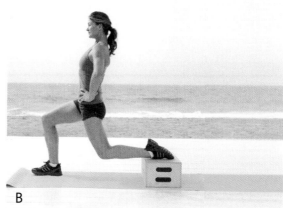

B

Mountain Climber

10 reps per side, alternating legs

> (A) Assume a full pushup position.
(B) Pull your right knee toward your chest, keeping your abs tight and hips level. Extend your right leg back to the starting position and repeat with your left leg.

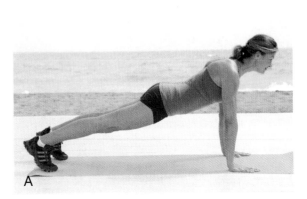

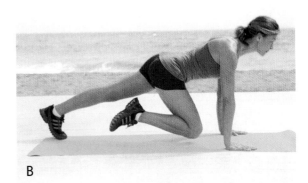

SUMMER-BODY WORKOUT Part 2: Fast Fat Burn

Vigorous cardio workouts like the one below have been shown to blast up to three times more thigh fat and five times more belly fat than moderate-intensity routines, getting you ready for shorts season in no time. You can do any type of cardio exercise for this workout: walking, jogging, cycling, swimming, or using a machine like the elliptical trainer.

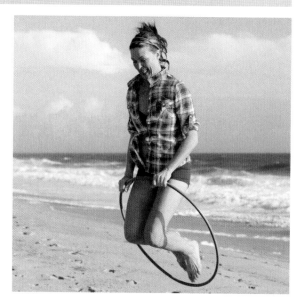

	Weeks 1 and 2	*Weeks 3 and 4*	*Weeks 5 and 6*	*Weeks 7 and 8*
Warmup	5 min, easy to moderate pace (can talk in full sentences)			
High-intensity interval	30 sec, fast (can talk in brief phrases only)	60 sec, fast	30 sec, very fast (don't want to talk)	60 sec, very fast
Recovery interval	60 sec, easy to moderate			
Reps	Do high-intensity and recovery intervals 6 times total			
Cooldown	5 min, moderate to easy			

Summary-Body Diet

You can slim down faster with our companion eating plan that curbs calories without making you hungry. The key is at least 25 grams a day of appetite-suppressing fiber, which has been shown

"WE SLIMMED DOWN AND LOST CELLULITE"

"I GOT A FRESH START"

Before: "My cellulite has gotten worse as I've gotten older, stopped exercising, and put on weight," says Liesa Goins, 35.

After: "I lost 8 pounds and 3 inches off my thighs. My cellulite has diminished, and I've tightened my belt two notches."

"I BUSTED MY PLATEAU"

Before: Avid exerciser Kathryn Townsend, 37, was struggling to take off her baby weight and reduce cellulite.

After: "I lost 10 pounds and 3 inches off my waist. My cellulite is almost gone, I can wear fitted clothing again, and my legs are toned."

"I SHRUNK MY 'MENO-POT' "

Before: Linda Mayerowitz, 62, really didn't have much weight to lose. But like many women her age, she was plagued by a widening waistline.

After: Her pants fit better, and she's at a healthy weight. "I lost 4 pounds and an inch off my waist."

to boost weight loss by an extra 2 to 3 pounds a month. At 1,800 calories a day, you'll have energy for exercise and keep your metabolism revved to make losing weight easier. (Drastically cutting calories can cause muscle loss, slow weight loss, and make cellulite look worse.) Here's a sample menu.

Breakfast: Latte and muffin: Mix $^2/_3$ cup warm 1 percent milk with strong coffee. Top a 2-ounce (Ping-Pong ball–size) bran muffin with 1 tablespoon peanut butter and serve with fruit salad ($^1/_2$ orange, peeled and chopped, and 1 kiwifruit, peeled and chopped).

401 calories, 10 g fiber

Lunch: Roast beef sandwich: Spread 2 slices 100 percent whole wheat bread with 1 tablespoon low-fat, low-sodium mayonnaise. Top with 2 thin slices roast beef (about 2 ounces) and 3 lettuce leaves. Serve with 12 baby carrots and 1 apple.

552 calories, 12 g fiber

Dinner: Pesto pasta: Toss $1^1/_2$ cups cooked linguine with 1 cup fresh diced tomatoes, 2 minced cloves garlic, $1^1/_2$ tablespoons pesto sauce, and 1 tablespoon grated Parmesan cheese. Serve with $1^1/_2$ cups cooked broccoli and $^1/_2$ cup lemon sorbet topped with $^1/_2$ cup blueberries.

656 calories, 14 g fiber

Snack: Veggies and dip: Slice 1 red bell pepper into strips, and dip it and 10 baby carrots into $^1/_3$ cup store-bought hummus.

197 calories, 15 g fiber

13

Beat Stress

FAT

Anxiety is a powerful biological trigger for weight gain, paving the way to diabetes. **Here's how to stop stressing—fast.**

For most of us, stress is a fact of life. Unfortunately, recent research reveals that it's also a fact of fat. "Even if you usually eat healthfully and exercise, chronic high stress can prevent you from losing weight—or even add pounds," says Pamela Peeke, MD, a *Prevention* advisor and the author of *Body for Life for Women.*

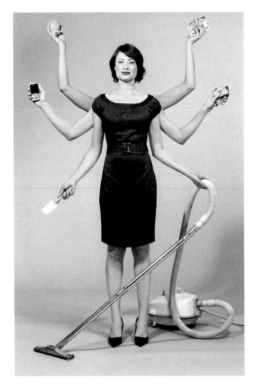

Here's what happens: Your body responds to all stress—physical or psychological—in exactly the same way. So every time you have a stressful day, your brain acts as though you're in physical danger and instructs your cells to release potent hormones. You get a burst of adrenaline, which taps stored energy so that you can fight or flee. At the same time, you get a surge of cortisol, which tells your body to replenish that energy even though you haven't used very many calories in your stressed-out state. This can make you hungry...very hungry. And your body keeps on pumping out that cortisol as long as the stress continues.

Sadly, few of us reach for carrot sticks in these situations.

"Instead we crave sweet, salty, and high-fat foods because they stimulate the brain to release pleasure chemicals that actually do reduce tension," explains Elissa S. Epel, PhD, a researcher on stress eating at the University of California, San Francisco. This soothing effect becomes addicting, so every time you're anxious, you reach for fattening foods.

In addition, with your adrenal glands pumping out cortisol, production of the muscle-building hormone testosterone slows down.

"Over time, this drop causes a decrease in your muscle mass, so you burn fewer calories," explains Shawn M. Talbott, PhD, author of *The Cortisol Connection*. "This occurs naturally as you age, but high cortisol levels accelerate the process."

Cortisol also encourages your body to store fat—especially visceral fat, which is particularly dangerous because it surrounds vital organs and releases fatty acids into your blood, raising cholesterol and insulin levels and paving the way for heart disease and diabetes.

Obviously, getting rid of all anxiety isn't an option. But by taking these seven steps to beat stress, you can get your cortisol levels and weight under control and improve your overall health at the same time.

Drop and Do 10

That's right, power out some pushups.

"Moving your muscles is an effective, instant stress reliever. It actually fools your body into thinking you're escaping the source of your stress," says Dr. Talbott. "Exercise makes your blood circulate more quickly, transporting the cortisol to your kidneys and flushing it out of your system."

But if pushups aren't practical, just flexing your hands or calf muscles will help move cortisol along, he explains. Even taking a stroll on your lunch break is beneficial. In one study, Dr. Talbott found that 18 minutes of walking three times per week can quickly lower the hormone's levels by 15 percent.

Go Slowly at Meals

Under stress, we tend to scarf down even healthy food, and research has linked this behavior to bigger portions and more belly fat. But Dr. Epel hypothesizes that slowing down, savoring each bite, and paying attention to feelings of fullness may lower cortisol levels as well as decrease the amount of food you eat, thereby shifting the distribution of fat away from the belly.

Stop Strict Dieting

It's ironic, but research shows that constant dieting can make cortisol levels rise by as much as 18 percent. In addition, when your cortisol levels spike, your blood sugar goes haywire, first rising, then plummeting. This makes you cranky and (you guessed it) ravenous. When your brain is deprived of sugar—its main fuel—self-control takes a nosedive, and your willpower doesn't stand a chance.

"The only way around this is to stop rigid dieting," advises Dr. Peeke. She suggests eating three healthful meals and two snacks spaced evenly throughout the day so that your blood sugar stays level: "You won't be hungry, you won't be stressed about being hungry, and you'll still drop the extra pounds."

Give In to Cravings

When stress drives you toward something sweet or salty, it's okay to yield a little.

"It's much better to indulge in a small way and cut off your cortisol response before it gets out of control," says Dr. Epel. "Have a piece of chocolate. You will feel better. Just stop at one."

If you have trouble restraining yourself, take precautions so you won't binge. Buy a single cookie when you're out instead of keeping a box at home, or keep them in the freezer so you have to wait for one to defrost.

Curtail Caffeine

Next time you're under duress, choose decaf. When you combine stress with caffeine, it raises cortisol levels more than stress alone.

In one study by the University of Oklahoma, consuming the equivalent of 2 1/2 to 3 cups of coffee while under mild stress boosted cortisol by about 25 percent—and kept it up for 3 hours. When subjects took 600 milligrams of caffeine (the equivalent of 6 cups of java) throughout the day, the hormone went up by 30 percent and stayed high all day long. You'll experience these effects even if your body is accustomed to a lot of lattes. And because high cortisol levels can contribute to stress eating, you might want to consider quitting caffeine altogether.

De-Stress Breakfast

Deficiencies in B vitamins, vitamin C, calcium, and magnesium are stressful to your body, leading to increased cortisol levels and food cravings, according to Dr. Talbott. But you can fight back by eating a breakfast that's high in these nutrients.

He suggests some OJ, a grapefruit, or a large handful of strawberries to supply vitamin C; 6 to 8 ounces of low-fat yogurt, which contains calcium and magnesium; and a whole grain bagel or toast with a bit of peanut butter. Whole grains are bursting with B vitamins, while peanut butter contains fatty acids that can decrease the production of stress hormones.

Sleep It Off

The most effective stress-reduction strategy of all: Get enough shut-eye.

"Your body perceives sleep deprivation as a major stressor," says Dr. Talbott. A University of Chicago study found that getting an average of 6 1/2 hours each night can increase cortisol, appetite, and weight gain. The National Sleep Foundation recommends 7 to 9 hours. As if that weren't enough, other research shows that lack of sleep also raises levels of ghrelin, which is a hunger-boosting hormone.

In one study, appetite—particularly for sweet and salty foods—increased by 23 percent in people who lacked sleep. The good news: A few nights of solid sleep can bring all this back into balance, and regularly getting enough sleep helps keep it there.

Says Dr. Talbott, "You'll eat less, and you'll feel better, too."

Stop Speed Eating

People who eat rapidly until they are full are three times more likely to be overweight than slow eaters, according to a study of more than 3,000 adults ages 30 to 69 that was conducted at Japan's Osaka University.

14

Shrink Your Belly Bloat
WITH FOOD

Here's what to add—and subtract—from your diet to **look and feel slimmer in less than a week.**

If belly bulge is sapping your summer-body confidence, don't despair. The reason for your puffy midsection may well be bloat, not fat. That's because one of the worst culprits in this problem—a slow digestive system—is common among women over age 40. However, exciting research now suggests that you can get your digestion moving and beat bloat with a few easy menu and lifestyle tweaks. Put all of these ideas into effect right now, and you should be feeling sexier and fitting more comfortably into your clothes in less than a week.

Eat These!

ADD: TWO KINDS OF FIBER

Why it beats bloat: Constipation distends your belly, and one easy way to get rid of it is by starting each morning with a breakfast cereal that guarantees your body a daily dose of fiber. This gets the digestive system moving within a day or so and keeps it that way. Based on a recent study of breakfast cereals, University of Toronto researchers say that consuming two kinds of fiber at once is most effective. The scientists found that study participants had an easier time staying regular when they ate a cereal that contained both insoluble fiber (from bran) and gel-like soluble fiber (from psyllium). The two types work together to pull water into the colon and speed up elimination, explains Joanne L. Slavin, PhD, a professor of food science and nutrition at the University of Minnesota in St. Paul. The result? You look and feel lighter.

THE NEWEST BELLY FLATTENER

Probiotics improve digestion, constipation, and bloating. Now research from Finland's University of Turku indicates that they may also cut belly fat by altering how we use and store energy. Yet according to the American Dietetic Association, only 20 percent of Americans have heard of probiotics. That's certain to change as companies roll out a new wave of products touting the gut-friendly bugs, giving consumers new ways to trim their tummies. Here, three of our favorites:

GoodBelly Probiotic Fruit Drink (120 calories per 8-ounce serving): Each serving boasts 20 billion live active probiotic cultures, similar to the amounts found in many yogurts.

Horizon Organic Cottage Cheese (120 calories per $\frac{1}{2}$ cup serving): This protein-packed snack will build muscle, maintain bones, and improve digestion.

Attune Granola Probiotic Wellness Bar (170 calories): Contains more than five times the probiotics found in yogurt and also packs prebiotics—fiber that feeds the bacteria in your gut. Find these products nationwide at grocery stores.

Good food fix: $1/3$ cup Kellogg's All-Bran Bran Buds each day

ADD: POTASSIUM-RICH FOODS

Why they beat bloat: Foods such as bananas and potatoes help your body get rid of excess water weight, minimizing your middle. The extra fluid is typically present because the two main minerals that control the amount of water in your body—potassium and sodium—have gotten out of balance. When your sodium level is too high, your tissues hold on to fluid. You can restore your sodium-potassium equilibrium by increasing your potassium intake to an optimum 4,700 milligrams per day. To do this, you need to eat about $4^1/2$ cups of produce daily, including the especially rich sources that are mentioned below. As you rebalance your system, you'll flush out the extra sodium along with the water. Presto: less puffiness.

Watch out, though. Food is a safe source of potassium, but supplements are not. They can cause potassium to build up in your body and potentially lead to abnormal heart rhythms and even heart attack, especially in people with kidney or heart problems, explains Leslie J. Bonci, RD, MPH, director of sports medicine nutrition at the Center for Sports Medicine at the University of Pittsburgh Medical Center.

Good food fixes: 1 medium baked potato with skin, 1 medium banana, 1 medium papaya, $1/2$ cup steamed edamame, $1/2$ cup tomato sauce, $1/2$ cup cooked spinach, 1 medium orange

ADD: YOGURT WITH PROBIOTICS

Why it beats bloat: Research published in *Alimentary Pharmacology & Therapeutics* reveals that an imbalance of bacteria in your gut can cause your digestive system to slow down and your belly to puff up. However, yogurts that contain live bacteria, otherwise known as probiotics, can help. Though researchers don't fully understand the mechanism, a study in the *Journal of the American Dietetic Association* found that the bacteria seem to tame tummy bloat by causing an improvement in intestinal mobility, thereby relieving constipation.

Good food fix: A daily 4-ounce container of low-fat or fat-free yogurt containing live, active cultures

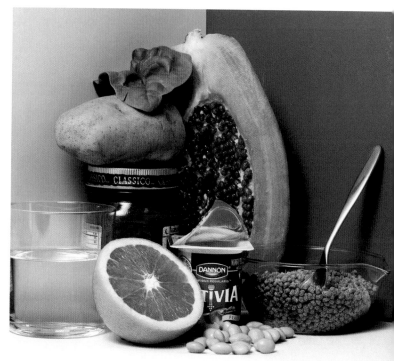

ADD: MORE FLUIDS

Why they beat bloat: Drinking enough liquid supports the other ways you're trying to flatten your tummy, according to Bonci. For example, she explains, when there's enough fluid present in your system, the dual-fiber cereal you have eaten is better able to pull liquid into your lower intestine and ease constipation. "Women who don't drink sufficient fluids can get that blown-up belly feeling, despite all their other efforts to get rid of it," warns Bonci.

How much fluid do you need? Getting rid of bloat means being well hydrated, so aim for at least 8 glasses of liquid each day, plus plenty of fluid-rich foods, such as fruits and vegetables. You can meet your quota with any liquid, including water, milk, juice, coffee, or tea—though not alcohol, which has a dehydrating effect on your system.

Good fluid fix: Tap water is an excellent option because it has no calories, salt, sugar, or additives. And it's free!

Don't Eat These!

SUBTRACT: SODIUM

Why it causes bloat: Sodium makes you retain water, puffing up your belly. Most of us eat more than twice as much sodium as we should—topping 3,400 milligrams a day rather than the recommended 1,500, according to the Centers for Disease Control and Prevention.

Good strategies: Stop salting your food at the table, and check for sodium on the labels of packaged foods, which provide about three-quarters of the daily intake for most women.

SUBTRACT: CANDY, SODA, AND GUM

Why they cause bloat: Once air from any source reaches your digestive system, you experience it as gas and a distended belly. Eating or drinking quickly, sipping through a straw, sucking on hard candy, and chewing gum can make you swallow air.

Good strategies: "When eating, chew slowly with your mouth closed," says Bonci. Trade carbonated drinks for flat ones, such as juice or water, and lose the gum and candies.

SUBTRACT: SUGAR ALCOHOLS

Why they cause bloat: We don't completely digest these low-calorie sweeteners (found in flavored waters and low-carb, diabetic, and sugar-free foods). Bacteria in the large intestine ferment them, causing gas and even diarrhea.

Good strategy: Check food labels to help avoid them; common sugar alcohols are sorbitol, mannitol, xylitol, and lactitol.

SUBTRACT: RAW PRODUCE

Why it causes bloat: Fresh fruits and vegetables are healthy, but they're also high-volume foods that take up room in your stomach, distending it.

Good strategies: Spread fresh produce consumption over the day so at any sitting, you're not eating more than one-third of the recommended daily total of $4^1/_2$ cups. You can also shrink produce by cooking it, creating a more compact serving, Bonci says.

Target Your Deepest

AB FAT

The key to a flat belly: **Engage hard-to-reach core muscles for ultrafast results.**

Hate crunches?

Say no more! Truth is, they do little to banish belly pooch anyway. For the fastest flattening, you need to target your deepest ab muscle: the transversus abdominis, also known as the TVA. Our exercise plan zeros in on the TVA and blasts the fat on top of it. Try it and you could drop a pound of fat a week, without dieting. Add our simple antibloat eating plan, and you could drop a size in 4 days!

Unlike other core muscles, the TVA runs horizontally and wraps around your midsection to suck in flab like a girdle and improve your posture so you look slimmer instantly. But most ab exercises miss the TVA because it's buried under the front and side torso muscles, and its actions are subtle. (You feel it engage when you sneeze.) According to research from Auburn University, moves that stabilize the midsection—such as the plank—are 34 percent more effective at targeting the TVA than traditional spine-flexing crunches. That's why you won't find a single situp in this workout.

Next, uncover those nicely toned abs with our fat-burning, customizable cardio interval routine. Australian research shows that this type of workout zaps belly fat faster than regular aerobic exercise.

For beach-ready abs in no time, combine these workouts with our antibloat eating plan to blast up to 7 pounds, nearly 5 inches from all over, and more than an inch off your belly in just 4 days.

Workout at a Glance

What you'll need: A stability ball, mat, and cloth belt (such as the one from your bathrobe)

3 days a week: Do the Tummy-Tucking Moves on nonconsecutive days, starting with 2 sets of 10 reps of each move (unless otherwise indicated).

3 alternate days: Follow the Belly-Blasting Intervals routine on page 128, using your choice of cardio activities.

For fastest results: Try our antibloat plan on page 127 and work up to a total of 3 sets of each Tummy-Tucking Move. Do 30 to 60 minutes of steady-paced cardio on these days, too, to burn even more calories.

The expert: Paul Frediani, master trainer at the Jewish Community Center health club in New York City and author of *Power Sculpt for Women*, designed this workout.

PART 1: TUMMY-TUCKING MOVES

For a more effective workout, start each session with the Ab Vacuum, which warms your TVA so you'll fully engage it throughout the routine.

Ab Vacuum

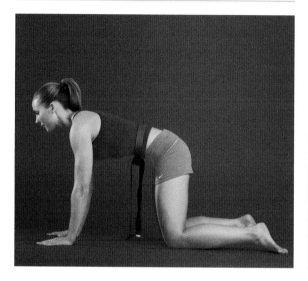

> Wrap the belt around your waist at belly button level, tying loose ends. Kneel with your hands on the floor below your shoulders, your knees beneath your hips, and your back flat. Breathe in deeply and expand your belly to press against the belt. Exhale, draw your belly button toward your spine (belt will loosen), and hold for 5 to 10 seconds (continue to breathe as you hold). Repeat 5 to 10 times.

Core Pulse

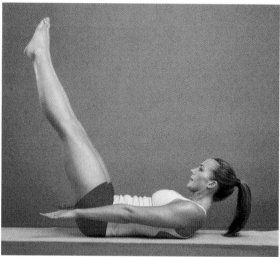

> Lie on your back with your arms at your sides, legs extended. Engage your abs and lift your head, shoulders, upper back, and arms a few inches off the floor. Inhale as you pulse your arms up and down an inch or two for a count of 5. Exhale, arms pulsing, for a count of 5. That's 1 rep.
> **Make it easier:** Do the move with your knees bent as much as 90 degrees.
> **Make it harder:** Lower your legs toward the floor, then pulse. The closer they are to the floor (without arching your back), the more challenging the move will be.

Elevated Plank

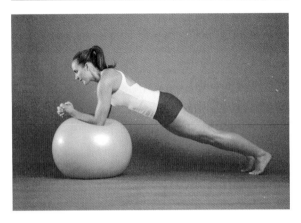

> Place your forearms on the ball, fingers interlaced, and extend your legs straight behind, supported on your toes. Exhale, pulling your belly button toward your spine, then hold for 30 to 60 seconds, with your back flat and body in a straight line. Rest for 30 seconds and repeat. Do 3 times.
> **Make it easier:** Do the plank with your forearms on the floor.
> **Make it harder:** From plank on the ball, alternate bringing your knees toward your chest for 10 reps per leg.

Double Reach

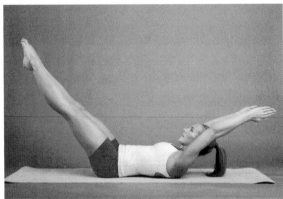

> Lie on your back, with your knees hugged to your chest and your head and shoulders lifted. Exhale, engage your abs, and extend your legs forward to about 45 degrees while reaching your arms back. Inhale and pull your knees and arms back into the start position.
> **Make it easier:** Keep your knees bent as you extend your legs forward.
> **Make it harder:** Lower your legs to just 2 to 3 inches off the floor.

Core Lunge

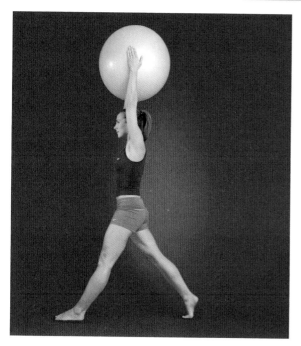
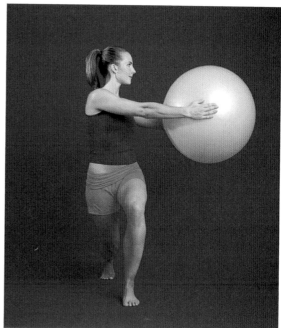

> Stand with your feet staggered, your left foot about 3 feet in front of the right, and hold the stability ball at chest level, arms extended. Inhale, engage your abs, and slowly lower, bending both knees to about 90 degrees (keep your front knee behind your toes). Exhale and, with control, stand up and raise the ball overhead, keeping your arms straight. Repeat, lowering the ball as you lunge.

> **Make it easier:** Do the move without holding the ball.
> **Make it harder:** From lunge position with your knees bent, rotate to the left, right, and back to center to complete 1 rep.

PART 1: TUMMY-TUCKING MOVES

Toe Dip

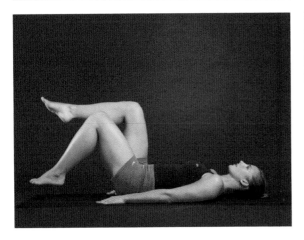

> Lie on your back with your legs over your hips and your knees bent to 90 degrees. Exhale, engage your abs, then slowly lower one foot almost to the floor, using your abs to keep your back from overarching. Return to the start position and switch legs.

> **Make it easier:** Plant one foot on the floor; lift and lower one leg at a time.

> **Make it harder:** Squeeze your legs together and lower both feet simultaneously.

Ball Balance

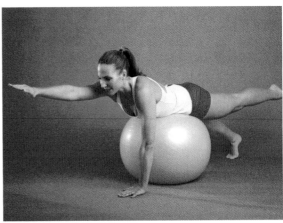

> Lie on the ball with your hands and toes on the floor. Exhale and pull your abs in to stabilize, then raise your right arm forward and your left leg back. Breathe and hold for 10 seconds, using your ab and back muscles to keep the ball steady and your body in a straight line, then lower. Repeat with the opposite arm and leg. Do five times on each side.

> **Make it easier:** Lift your arm for only 5 reps, then repeat with the opposite leg. Switch sides and repeat.

> **Make it harder:** Hold the raised position as you write the alphabet in the air with your extended arm. Switch sides and repeat.

Fast Results! Eat to Beat Bloat

This 1,200-calorie 4-day diet, designed by a registered dietitian, quickly nixes bloat for fast flattening. It doesn't burn fat, though, so don't skip the workouts. (Do them about 2 hours after a meal for maximum energy.) Drink plenty of water throughout, and after 4 days, continue with a 1,600-calorie plan, such as the Flat Belly Diet (www.prevention.com/flatbellydiet).

BREAKFAST

1 cup unsweetened cornflakes or Rice Krispies, or 1 packet Cream of Wheat

1 cup fat-free milk

1/4 cup roasted or raw unsalted sunflower seeds

1/2 cup unsweetened applesauce, 4 ounces canned pineapple in juice, or 2 tablespoons raisins or 2 dried plums

Per serving: 396 calories, 16 g protein, 41 g carbohydrates, 6 g fiber, 21 g fat, 2 g saturated fat, 4 mg cholesterol, 213 mg sodium

LUNCH

4 ounces organic deli turkey, rolled up, or 3 ounces chunk light tuna in water

1 piece light string cheese

1 pint fresh grape tomatoes, or 1 cup steamed or microwaved baby carrots

Per serving: 215 calories, 9 g protein, 27 g carbohydrates, 3 g fiber, 3 g fat, 2 g saturated fat, 61 mg cholesterol, 825 mg sodium

SMOOTHIE

1 cup fat-free milk and 1 cup frozen unsweetened blueberries (or strawberries or peaches), processed in a blender for 1 minute

Transfer to a glass and stir in 1 tablespoon cold-pressed organic flaxseed oil.

Per serving: 263 calories, 9 g protein, 27 g carbohydrates, 3 g fiber, 15 g fat, 1 g saturated fat, 5 mg cholesterol, 104 mg sodium

DINNER

3 ounces chicken or turkey breast, or 4 ounces tilapia, grilled

1/2 cup roasted red potatoes drizzled with 1 teaspoon olive oil,* or 1/2 cup brown rice

1 cup fresh mushrooms or yellow squash sautéed in 1 teaspoon olive oil,** or 1 cup fresh or frozen green beans, steamed

Per serving: 290 calories, 30 g protein, 13 g carbohydrates, 2 g fiber, 13 g fat, 2 g saturated fat, 72 mg cholesterol, 73 mg sodium

*If you choose this item, steam or microwave your vegetables only to limit your oil intake.

**If you choose this item, have the brown rice instead of the potatoes to limit your oil intake.

PART 2: BELLY-BLASTING INTERVALS

Women who did just 20 minutes of interval training lost 3 pounds from their bellies during a 15-week study. Here's a fun, equipment-free version you can do in your living room, backyard, or local park. You can also swap your favorite style of cardio (like walking, jogging, swimming, or cycling) into the chart below, alternating 20 seconds at a vigorous intensity with 40-second recovery bouts at a moderate pace. Whatever activity you pick, focus on pulling your belly button to your spine to target your TVA throughout the routine.

Time	What to Do
0:00–3:00	March in place to warm up (level 4-5*).
3:00–3:20	Highs and Lows (level 8-9): Stand with feet hip-width apart, hands at sides. Bend knees and squat down to touch floor, then reach up overhead, rising onto toes, and lower to repeat.
3:20–4:00	March in place (level 5-6).
4:00–4:20	Jumping Jacks (level 8-9): Jump, landing with feet wide, arms overhead; jump again, bringing feet together, arms at sides.
4:20–5:00	March in place (level 5-6).
5:00–5:20	Knee Pulls (level 8-9): Balance on right leg, knee bent slightly, and raise left knee forward to hip height, then immediately extend it behind you, touching toes to floor, and repeat. Bend arms and swing them in opposition. Switch legs the next time you do this exercise.
5:20–6:00	March in place (level 5-6).
6:00–6:20	Claps (level 8-9): Hop and lift one knee at a time toward chest as you alternate clapping hands under the elevated leg and overhead.
6:20–7:00	March in place (level 5-6).

Make Small Changes to Take Off

BIG POUNDS

Quadruple your weight loss by making one easy tweak per week to your routine.

If you've been diagnosed with diabetes, it's a good bet that your doctors have suggested losing weight. But you can forget the deprivation diet and marathon workouts. New research shows that taking baby steps—not giant leaps—is the best way to get lasting results.

A study published in the *Annals of Behavioral Medicine* found that participants who made one small, potentially permanent change in their food choices and/or physical activity each week (such as drinking one less can of soda or walking 5 more minutes each day) during a 4-month program got great results, compared with those who followed traditional guidelines for calorie restrictions and physical activity: They lost more than twice as much belly fat, $2^1/_2$ more inches off their waistlines, and about four times more weight.

"When you focus on just a couple of small changes at a time, you begin to ingrain some healthy habits that last for a lifetime, rather than trying an all-or-nothing approach that more often than not fails because it's too hard to follow," says Lesley Lutes, PhD, an assistant professor in the department of psychology at East Carolina University in Greenville.

We've uncovered 11 simple steps (with proven results) to help you move more, eat less, and look and feel better than ever. Add just one or two a week to your regular routine, and you can lose nearly 3 inches off your waistline and be about 10 pounds lighter in a few short months.

Even better: Once these healthy habits become second nature, they'll benefit you for a lifetime.

Pick Up a Pen after Every Meal

Mindlessly munch on a bag of chips and you could easily polish off the whole thing; write down how much you've eaten and you're more likely to practice portion control.

Keeping a food log helps you control extra calories in two ways: by giving you a plain old reality check (I just ate 30 minutes ago!) and making you aware that what you're putting in your mouth will soon be recorded for posterity.

In a recent study, people who kept a food journal lost twice as much weight as those who didn't. When they combined their writing with a moderate diet and exercise plan, they lost an average of 13 pounds in 6 months. Journaling also gives you insight into your eating habits, explains Dr. Lutes. Do you skip meals? Eat the same during the week as on the weekend? Binge when you're feeling stressed?

"Knowing your routine helps you figure out what changes are right for you," she adds. Make it simple by tracking yourself online at www.prevention.com/healthtracker.

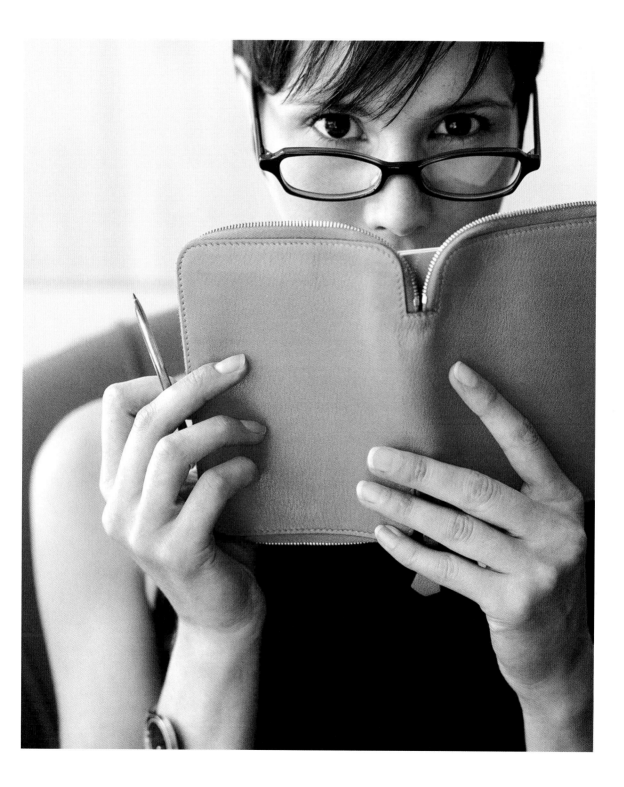

Nine Easy Swaps That Save Loads of Calories

Shaving some calories from every meal, snack, or side dish is one of the easiest ways to reduce your overall intake. To lose $1/2$ to 1 pound a week, aim to cut 250 to 500 calories a day by making two or three of these swaps.

Swap	Save
1 can regular soda for 1 bottle water	100 calories
Small french fries for apple slices	270 calories
1 c chocolate ice cream for $1/2$ c chocolate ice cream with $1/2$ c sliced strawberries	115 calories
Big Mac for regular hamburger	290 calories
$1/2$ c granola for $3/4$ c high-fiber cereal	110 calories
1 Tbsp mayo for 1 tsp mustard on sandwich	100 calories
1 large ($4^1/2$-inch) bagel for 2 slices light whole grain bread	269 calories
1 small bag (1 oz) pretzels for 2 c air-popped popcorn	47 calories
2 slices pizza for 1 slice cheese pizza plus $1^1/2$ c mixed salad with 1 Tbsp low-fat dressing	229 calories

Skip through the Commercials

Get off your duff and move during your favorite TV shows. Skip, dance, go up and down some stairs, run in place—anything that gets your heart rate up so you feel somewhat breathless, says Geralyn Coopersmith, senior national manager at Equinox Fitness. Do it for each 2-minute break (forget the TiVo) during a typical 2-hour TV night and you'll burn an extra 270 calories a day, which can translate into a 28-pound weight loss in a year.

Limit High-Fat Foods to One per Week

Tag the high-fat, high-calorie foods that are your favorites and gradually downshift.

"If you're eating six of these foods a week, try to go down to five," says Dr. Lutes. Each week, drop another until you're at no more than one or two. At the same time, add in a good-for-you choice like baby carrots, sautéed broccoli, oranges, or other fresh fruits and veggies.

Sign Up for Healthy E-Newsletters

One recent study from Kaiser Permanente found that people who received weekly e-mails about diet and fitness for 16 weeks substantially increased their levels of physical activity and intake of healthy foods such as fruits and vegetables while cutting back on trans and saturated fats.

We can help: Go to www.prevention. com/newsletters and sign up for our weekly newsletters *Eat Up, Slim Down* and *Walk Off the Weight.*

Walk 5 Minutes More Every Day

In Dr. Lutes's pilot study, increasing daily activity levels by just a few minutes at a time helped participants lose weight. Eventually your goal should be to do at least 30 minutes of physical activity a day (burning off about 120 extra calories daily, or $12\frac{1}{2}$ pounds a year), but it doesn't have to be all at once.

Here are some simple ways to get moving.

- Walk around the perimeter of the grocery store at least once before heading toward the items you need.

- Move in place whenever you're talking on the telephone.

- Go through or around the entire shopping mall instead of parking near the store you need.

- Take a walk around the block at lunch and after dinner.

Strength-Train in Minibursts

Basic body-weight exercises such as squats and pushups are a simple way to build more metabolism-revving muscle in minutes, and research shows that they're just as effective as hitting the gym.

"Your muscles don't know the difference between working against your body's own resistance and on a fancy piece of equipment," says *Prevention* advisor Wayne L. Westcott, PhD, fitness research director at Quincy College in Massachusetts. "The one rule to follow is that each exercise should fatigue your muscles within 60 to 90 seconds."

Try this miniworkout: Do 10 reps each of knee pushups, squats, crunches, lunges, and chair dips. Then gradually increase the number of reps it takes for your muscles to feel fully fatigued.

Climb Three Extra Flights of Stairs Daily

Have a choice between riding and climbing? Including 2 to 3 minutes of stair-climbing per day—covering about three to five floors—can burn enough calories to eliminate the average American's annual weight gain of 1 to 2 pounds a year.

It's also good for more than just your

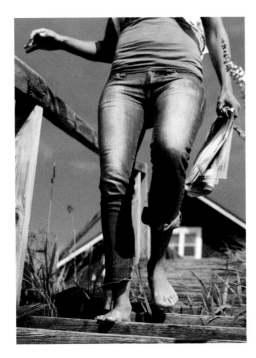

Find the latest pedometer styles, including one you can toss in a purse, at www.prevention.com/pedometer.

Brown-Bag It at Least Once a Week

You'll save thousands of calories (not to mention hundreds of dollars) over the course of a year. Consider this: A premade chicken Caesar wrap from a chain restaurant has about 610 calories, more than 40 percent of which come from fat, as well as 1,440 milligrams of sodium, which is more than half the recommended daily amount.

Make your own with presliced deli chicken breast on whole wheat bread with light mayo and romaine for about 230 calories. You'll cut almost 400 calories and about 520 milligrams of sodium, which leaves room for a side salad and could still add up to a 28-pound weight loss after a year.

"When you make and eat your own food, you not only control the quality and portion sizes but also reduce the amount of sugar, salt, and fat that you're consuming, which can be significantly higher in restaurant fare," says Ashley Koff, RD, a nutrition consultant based in Los Angeles.

waistline: Men who climbed more than 70 flights of stairs a week had 18 percent lower mortality rates than those who climbed fewer than 20 flights a week, according to one Harvard study. Start with just a couple of flights a day; if you're already a dedicated climber, aim to add three more flights to your daily trek.

Take a Pedometer Wherever You Go

Just as you wouldn't leave home without your cell phone, make a pedometer a must-have accessory. Research shows that pedometer users take nearly 2,500 more steps a day (more than 1 mile, or about 100 calories) than nonusers. Over a year, that's enough to burn off about 10 pounds.

Doing Errands? Obey the 1-Mile Rule

Americans use their cars for two-thirds of all trips that are less than 1 mile and

89 percent of all trips that are 1 to 2 miles, yet each additional hour you spend driving is associated with a 6 percent increase in obesity.

Burn calories instead of gas by following this rule: If your errands are less than 1 mile away, vow to walk them at a brisk pace instead of driving. Or park where you can run several errands within a mile instead of moving your car each time. Walk every day, and you'll be 13 to 17 pounds lighter next year.

Take 10 Minutes to Eat a Treat

Try this strategy to reduce cravings permanently: Portion out one serving of your favorite treat, taking a minute to smell it, look at it, and think about it.

Take one small bite. Chew slowly, moving it around your mouth and focusing on the texture and taste, then swallow. Ask yourself whether you want another bite or if that satisfied you. If you still want more, repeat, this time chewing 20 times. Continue this eating exercise for as long as you want or until you finish the serving (it should take about 10 minutes).

"When you take the time to slow down and be more mindful of what something really tastes like, you'll feel more satisfied," says Dr. Lutes. "Many of our participants told us that after a while, they didn't enjoy the treat as much as they thought they would, or they were content after just a couple of bites and were better able to stop eating when they were satisfied."

For more easy ways to lose weight, go to www.prevention.com/smallchanges.

MOVE

Exercise is often the best prescription

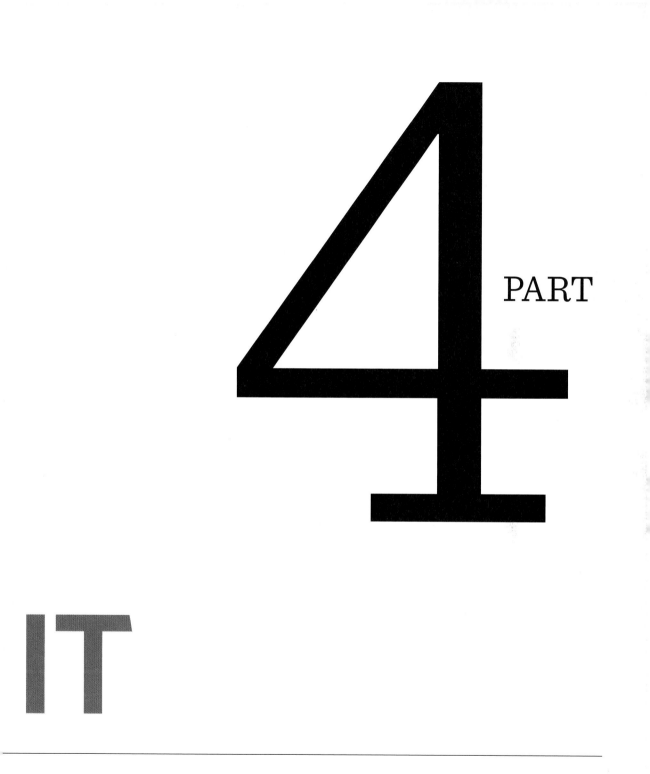

PART

4

IT

for losing weight—and feeling great.

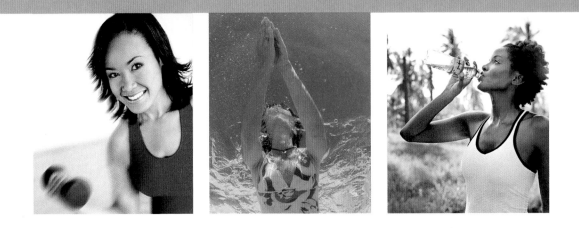

EXERCISE
Medical Breakthroughs

Researchers discovered that even one exercise session lowers insulin levels. That's great reason to get moving—today! For most people, exercise is perfectly safe. But we recommend that you talk with your doctor first if you've had a heart attack, asthma, heart disease, liver or kidney disease, arthritis, osteoporosis, dizziness or balance problems, chest or joint pain, or persistent pain or other problems from a joint or muscle injury; or if you take medication for a chronic medical condition.

MAKE EXERCISE STICK

Need a reason to start working out again—and the motivation to keep at it this time? Forget weight loss and focus on quality of life, advises Michelle Segar, PhD, at the University of Michigan's Institute for Research on Women and Gender in Ann Arbor. She found that women ages 40 to 60 who exercised with a goal of overall well-being were 34 percent more likely to stick with it than those interested only in losing weight. Women who exercised to maintain their weight also kept at it more than those who felt pressured to shed pounds.

BIG DAY? PUT FITNESS FIRST

Feeling mentally exhausted can sabotage your workouts. Welsh researchers found that brain drain saps physical energy, making you more likely to quit early. Adults who exercised after a mentally challenging 90-minute test fatigued 15 percent faster than those who watched a 90-minute video about trains before working out. Scientists suspect that challenges to the mind and muscles tap the same area of the brain that's linked to your perception of physical effort. Work out in the morning of a busy day to blast more fat and improve your focus all day.

MAKE OVER YOUR HEALTH

Good news for your busiest days: Just 3 minutes of exercise can yield significant health benefits, according to a recent Scottish study. Adults who did six 30-second sprints on an exercise bike (resting 4 minutes in between) improved their bodies' ability to metabolize blood sugar by nearly 25 percent after six sessions—enough to lower their risks of diabetes and heart disease. Try it while watching your favorite TV show. Run up and down the stairs or do jumping jacks during an ad (most are about 30 seconds); rest until the next commercial break.

GET A HEALTHIER BODY IN ONE WORKOUT

Just a single exercise session increases the rate of fat burning and muscle building while lowering insulin levels, a University of Michigan study of obese women found. Researchers tested 90-minute workouts; coauthor Jeffrey Horowitz, PhD, has begun studying 45-minute exercise sessions and thinks that shorter stints might yield similar benefits.

TRICK YOURSELF THIN

Need motivation to stick with a strength-training regimen? Try starting small, suggests a new Elon University study. Researchers found that exercisers who worked minor muscle groups first (like the biceps and calves) and then moved up to bigger muscle groups (like the back and quadriceps) built up less muscle-tiring lactic acid than those who did the reverse order, allowing them to complete more reps in each set for speedier firming. Plus, they reported that their workouts felt easier, and they finished in better moods.

The percentage of morning exercisers who stick to their workouts, according to the Mollen Clinic in Phoenix:

75

PREVENT SUGAR DAMAGE

Here's motivation to pencil in an a.m. workout when the evening's festivities are going to include sweets: A Washington University School of Medicine study found that exercise might protect your heart long after you step off the treadmill. Sugary snacks cause blood vessels to lose their elasticity temporarily, which over time increases heart disease risk, but physical activity can help: When each subject was given a candy bar and soda 17 hours after doing an hour of moderate-intensity cardio, the exercisers were able to pump 28 percent more blood than those who'd rested and eaten the same sugar-laden meal.

TAKE AN EXERCISE BREAK

Another reason to exercise during your lunch break: An easy 30-minute bike ride or stroll after eating may control insulin and blood sugar as well as drugs can, a Norwegian study found. Improved insulin response means fewer blood sugar spikes that encourage your body to pack away extra fat and raise your risk of heart disease, diabetes, and obesity. Further research is needed to determine the best exercise dose, but scientists suggest that even a 10- to 15-minute session could be beneficial.

Just 2.5 hours of exercise a week could bring the following amazing benefits:

- Almost eliminate type 2 diabetes (up to 91 percent less cases)

- Reduce heart attacks by one-third

- Prevent 285,000 deaths from heart disease in the United States alone

DIVE INTO LONGEVITY

For the ultimate antiaging workout, grab a pair of goggles. South Carolina researchers followed 40,547 adults ages 20 to 90 for more than 3 decades and discovered that swimmers—regardless of age—were about 50 percent less likely to die during the study than were sofa sitters, walkers, and runners. Scientists speculate that water-based workouts are tops for lifelong fitness, thanks to their low injury risk and built-in full-body toning, combined with joint-friendly cardio.

EXERCISERS: SKIP THESE SUPPLEMENTS

News flash: Popping vitamin C and E supplements may counteract your workout's ability to protect against diabetes. In a new study, insulin sensitivity did not improve in exercisers given 1,000 milligrams of vitamin C and 400 IU of vitamin E daily (the dose in typical drugstore brands), while those who did the same workouts without extra antioxidants significantly improved their ability to process blood sugar over 4 weeks. Supplements may prevent the body from producing its own antioxidants, according to researchers, hampering exercise's disease-fighting benefits. Get these vitamins naturally from produce, nuts, seeds, and oils.

Move More:
HERE'S WHY

Exercise makes you sharper, happier, and healthier.
Get ready to transform your life!

Have you ever vowed to ring in a new year by starting to exercise—only to end up too busy, tired, or achy? The right motivation can make you 70 percent more likely to keep it up for the long haul, reports the American College of Sports Medicine. But focusing only on weight loss can cut your odds of success by more than half, according to researchers. A better inspiration: the amazing health rewards you get by being active. A stronger heart and lower cancer risk are two well-known benefits. Here are more benefits that are guaranteed to motivate.

Improve Language Skills A single treadmill session can make you brainier. In a study by Germany's University of Muenster, exercisers who ran just two 3-minute sprints, with a 2-minute break in between, learned new words 20 percent faster than those who rested. Getting your heart pumping increases blood flow, delivering more oxygen to your noggin. It also spurs new growth in the areas of the brain that control multitasking, planning, and memory.

Do this: Add a bout of exercise, such as running up and down the stairs, before you try to memorize anything—say, Spanish phrases for your trip to Mexico.

Get All-Natural Pain Relief It might seem counterintuitive, but rest isn't necessarily best for reducing pain and stiffness in the knees, shoulders, back, or neck. Healthy adults who did aerobic activity consistently had 25 percent less musculoskeletal pain than their couch-bound peers, according to Stanford senior research scientist Bonnie Bruce, DrPH.

Exercise releases endorphins, which are the body's natural pain reliever, and it might make you less vulnerable to tiny tears in muscles and tendons.

Staying active can also provide relief for chronic conditions such as arthritis: In a University of North Carolina at Chapel Hill study, arthritis sufferers experienced 25 percent less pain and 16 percent less stiffness after 6 months of low-impact exercise such as balance and strengthening moves. Most people start to feel improvement within a few weeks, observes study author Leigh F. Callahan, PhD, an associate professor of medicine at the school.

Do this: Practice yoga or tai chi twice a week; both activities increase flexibility and range of motion and reduce pain.

Be Happier at Work An active lifestyle may help you check off extra items on your to-do list, according to a study from the University of Bristol in the United Kingdom. On days staffers participated in on-site fitness activities, they reported thinking more clearly, getting more done, and interacting more effectively with colleagues.

You'll be less likely to miss work because of illness, too. Research shows that people who participate in vigorous leisure-time physical activity (such as jogging or bicycling) just once or twice a

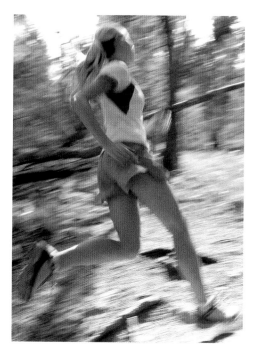

benefits stand the test of time: A Harvard study of swimmers found that those over age 60 were as satisfied sexually as those decades younger.

Do this: Try 20 minutes of aerobics before a romantic evening. To feel good naked anytime, walk or do yoga daily.

Lower Dental Bills Flossing and brushing, it turns out, are not the only keys to a healthy smile, advises Mohammad Al-Zahrani, DDS, PhD, a former associate professor at Case Western Reserve University in Cleveland. Exercise plays an important role, too. In his recent study, Dr. Al-Zahrani discovered that adults who did 30 minutes of moderate activity five or more times a week were 42 percent less likely to suffer from periodontitis, which is a gum disease that's more likely to develop as you get older. Working out may thwart periodontitis the same way it does heart disease—by lowering levels of inflammation-causing C-reactive protein in the blood.

Do this: In addition to staying active, get a twice-yearly dental cleaning—or more often if your dentist says you are at high risk for gum disease.

Slash Cold Risk by 33 Percent Moderate exercise doesn't just rev your metabolism. It boosts your immune system, too, helping your body fight off cold bugs and other germs. Women ages 50 to 75 who did 45 minutes of cardio, 5 days a week, had a third as many colds as those who did once-weekly stretching sessions, a University of Washington study found.

Do this: Stay active, but don't overdo it.

week take about half the sick time of those who are more sedentary.

Do this: Sign up for workplace fitness classes. None on-site? Ask human resources to designate a room for a noontime yoga session, using DVD or videotape instruction. Or recruit co-workers to go for a lunch-hour power walk.

Feel Sexy at Any Size A good workout practically ensures a better body image. A Pennsylvania State University study found that women ages 42 to 58 felt more attractive after 4 months of walking or doing yoga even if they didn't lose weight.

Exercise can also put you in the mood for love by increasing blood flow to the genitals. University of Washington research found that just one 20-minute cycling workout enhanced sexual arousal in women by up to 169 percent. And the

PACK A SNACK

If you have type 2 diabetes and use insulin, ask your doctor how much exercise you can tolerate before you need to replenish your store of carbohydrates. Carry a healthy snack (an apple or a handful of trail mix) with you on your walks for just this purpose.

More than 90 minutes of vigorous exercise, such as running, most days might actually reduce immunity.

Reach the Deep-Sleep Zone Say good night to poor sleep. Women ages 60 and older who walked or danced for at least an hour four times a week woke up half as often and slept an average 48 minutes more a night than sedentary women did, according to a study in the journal *Sleep Medicine*. That is good news for the many women who toss and turn more as they get older. As you age, sleep patterns start shifting, so you spend more of the night in lighter sleep phases, explains Shawn D. Youngstedt, PhD, an assistant professor of exercise science at the University of South Carolina in Columbia.

Do this: Aim to exercise for at least half an hour, even if it's after a long day. Evidence suggests that for most people, light to moderate activity in the evening won't disturb sleep, though trial and error will tell you what works for you.

Beat Bloating The next time you feel puffy around the middle, resist the urge to stay put. A study from Spain's Autonomous University of Barcelona suggests that mild physical activity clears gas and alleviates bloating. That's because increasing your heart rate and breathing stimulates the natural contractions of the intestinal muscles, helping to prevent constipation and gas buildup by expediting digestion.

Do this: Walk or pedal lightly on a bike until you feel better.

See Clearly What's good for your heart is good for your eyes. An active lifestyle can cut your risk of age-related macular degeneration by up to 70 percent, according to a *British Journal of Ophthalmology* study of 4,000 adults. This incurable disease makes reading, driving, and seeing fine details difficult, and it's the most common cause of blindness after age 60.

Do this: Keep active by walking at least 12 blocks (about a mile) a day, and wear UVA- and UVB-blocking sunglasses during outdoor activities all year long.

Enjoy Instant Energy If you're among the 50 percent of adults who report feeling tired at least 1 day a week, skip the java and go for a walk. University of Georgia researchers who analyzed 70 different studies concluded that moving your body increases energy and reduces fatigue. Regular exercise boosts certain fatigue-fighting brain chemicals such as norepinephrine and dopamine, which pep you up, and serotonin, a mood enhancer.

Do this: Take a 20-minute stroll for a quick pick-me-up, or aim for 40 minutes of activity daily for a sustained lift.

18

Be a Little GRACEFUL

Good coordination helps you feel young, strong, and healthy for life. **Here's how to stay light on your feet.**

S lips, trips, and falls are great fodder for sitcom jokes, but as we age, falls are no laughing matter. In fact, they're one of the most serious medical problems facing older people. This is especially important for people with diabetes, who might have difficulty healing if they're injured in a fall.

Grace is a crucial survival skill, but it's also perishable. Ever so gradually after we hit 30, muscles we use to stand tall weaken. The length of our strides shortens, the pace of our steps slows, and vision—critical to coordination—becomes fuzzier. Even menopause can make our gaits a tad more wobbly.

"Aging, however, isn't the only reason people lose their sense of stability," says A. Lynn Millar, PhD, a professor of physical therapy at Andrews University in Berrien Springs, Michigan. "Balance is really 'use it or lose it.' You can maintain it if you stay active."

How well we keep our balance now, in

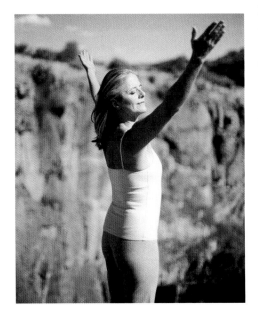

midlife, can protect us from what lies ahead: One in three adults over age 65 takes a serious tumble each year. Avoiding falls means a longer life: About 20 percent of women who fracture a hip become permanently disabled, and another 20 percent die within a year. In fact, health problems linked to hip fractures result in more women's deaths each year than breast cancer does.

But an enhanced sense of stability doesn't just help protect you from future falls. There are immediate health benefits— better mobility, fewer injuries, greater capacity to push yourself harder during workouts—that increase overall fitness, points out Fabio Comana, an exercise physiologist with the American Council on Exercise.

The problem is that people are often unaware that their coordination is slipping. While there are hallmarks of clumsiness—such as poor handwriting and banged-up shins and knees—even naturally agile people need to work to boost balance with age. (To see where you stand, try "Test Your Balance" moves.)

"Balance is a separate system, just like strength or flexibility. You can improve it if you continue to challenge it," says Edward R. Laskowski, MD, codirector of the Mayo Clinic Sports Medicine Center in Rochester, Minnesota.

TEST YOUR BALANCE

Try these three simple exercises to see how balanced you are.

1. Stand with your feet together, anklebones touching, and your arms folded across your chest; then close your eyes. Have someone time you: Though it's normal to sway a little, you should be able to stand for 60 seconds without moving your feet. Next, place one foot directly in front of the other and close your eyes. You should be able to stand for at least 38 seconds on each side.

2. Stand on one foot and bend the other knee, lifting the nonsupporting foot off the floor without letting it touch the standing leg. (Do this in a doorway so you can grab the sides if you start to fall.) Repeat with your eyes closed. People age 60 and younger can typically hold the pose for about 29 seconds with their eyes open, 21 seconds with their eyes closed. People age 61 and older: 22 seconds with eyes open, 10 seconds with eyes closed.

3. Stand on the ball of one foot with your hands on your hips, and place the nonsupporting foot against the inside of the knee of the standing leg. Raise your heel off the floor and hold the pose—you should be able to do so for 25 seconds.

How did you do? If you scored below average on any of these measures, boost your balance with the moves from this story and more at www.prevention.com/balance.

Here are six strategies to help strengthen the core and lower-body muscles that keep you steady on your feet.

Stand on one leg: Try to do this while you are washing the dishes, suggests Dr. Laskowski. When you can hold the pose for 30 seconds on each side, stand on a less stable surface, such as a couch cushion. To increase the challenge even more, do it with your eyes closed.

Take a tai chi class: A recent study of tai chi practitioners in their midsixties found that on measures of stability, most scored around the 90th percentile of the American Fitness Standards. Yoga works, too: According to Temple University research, women 65 and older who took twice-weekly yoga classes for 9 weeks increased ankle flexibility and showed more confidence in walking. That last part is important, says lead researcher Jinsup Song, DPM, PhD, "because when people are fearful of losing balance, they tend to do less to challenge themselves."

That fear doesn't plague only the elderly: A Howard University study found that among those 65 and older, 22 percent had already become fearful of falling.

Walk heel to toe: The same sobriety field test that cops give drunk drivers also improves balance. Take 20 steps forward, heel to toe. Then walk backward, with toe to heel, in a straight line.

Do squats: Sturdy legs can help prevent a stumble from turning into a fall, explains Comana. To build quads, start

KNEES HURT? TRY TAI CHI

Thinking about trying tai chi? A Tufts Medical Center study found that adults with knee osteoarthritis—the most common joint disease in midlife—saw up to three times greater improvement in both pain and joint function from biweekly hour-long tai chi sessions than did those who attended stretching and wellness classes. Experts say the flowing, meditative movements tone the muscles surrounding joints, enhance body awareness to reduce risk of injury, and improve alignment.

with a simple squat: With your feet hip-width apart, bend your knees and hips and slowly lower yourself as if sitting in a chair behind you. Keep your arms straight out, abs tight, back straight, and knees above shoelaces. Stop when your thighs are parallel to the floor (or as close as you can get), then contract your glutes as you stand back up. Aim for 3 sets of 10, with a 1-minute break after each.

Practice the force: It takes muscle strength to get out of a chair, but it takes muscle force to do it quickly.

"That force—the ability to get your leg in the right place in a nanosecond—is important in preventing falls," says Comana. We lose muscle force faster than strength, and according to new research, it takes older women longer to build it back up.

Try this move: Instead of gingerly rising from a chair, once in a while leap out of it so forcefully that you need to take a few running steps after you do so. (You can use your arms to gain momentum.)

"The explosiveness of that action builds power," says Comana. Side-to-side and back-to-front muscle movements have the same effect, such as when you play tennis or basketball.

Balance on a wobble board: It's one of a few gym gizmos designed to challenge your stability. Stand on the board with your feet shoulder-width apart, abs tight, and rock forward and back and side to side for a minute at a time. (Hold a chair for support, if needed.) Work up to 2 minutes, without holding on or letting the edges of the device touch the floor.

"Keep injecting novelty into your routine," says Dr. Millar. "Push yourself to try something new, and you'll boost both balance and overall health."

Bonus Balance Tip

Sleep more than 7 hours a night.
Sleep deprivation slows reaction time, and a study at California Pacific Medical Center shows that it's also directly related to falls. Researchers tracked nearly 3,000 older women and found that those who typically slept between 5 and 7 hours each night were 40 percent more likely to fall than those who slept longer.

Get Fit and Firm
AT HOME

Fight diabetes from your living room with our top DVD picks, plus three targeted plans to slim you down fast—whatever your level.

There's proof that the best workout in town starts by pressing "play." A new study has found that doing fitness DVDs can burn a whopping 480 calories an hour. We sweated through more than 40 new releases to bring you our five faves: workouts that are effective, easy to follow, and fun. Whether you want to drop a size, shrink stubborn belly fat, or just start exercising, we have the plan for you.

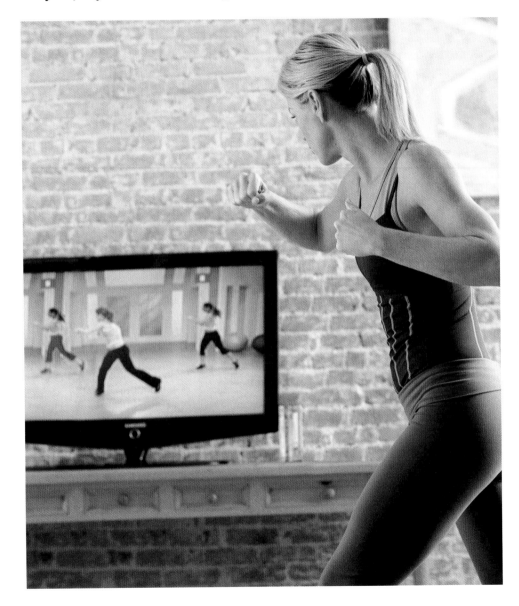

Here are five *Prevention*-tested DVDs we love. Pick just one, mix and match, or follow our customized plans designed to help you achieve your fitness goal.

10-Minute Solution: Quick Tummy Toners

Focus: Targeted toning

Why we love it: The five fast, doable routines—from calorie-torching standing exercises to mat-based whittlers—beat boredom and firm your abs from every angle.

You'll need: Yoga mat

6-Minute Quick Blast: Total Body Calorie Blast

Focus: Cardio and toning

Why we love it: Whether you have 6 minutes or an hour, you'll get a heart-pumping cardio blast plus intense sculpting to reshape trouble zones like the butt, thighs, and abs.

You'll need: Yoga mat, dumbbells

Prevention: Kick-Start Your Metabolism

Focus: Cardio and toning

Why we love it: *Prevention* fitness pro Chris Freytag will teach you to punch, jab, and kick your way to a firmer body—no experience needed. You'll melt up to 680 calories an hour while having a blast.

You'll need: Yoga mat, dumbbells

Exhale: Core Fusion Pilates Plus

Focus: All-over toning

Why we love it: Carefully controlled movements target each muscle group with laserlike precision. Gentle stretches end each segment to ease your body and mind.

You'll need: Yoga mat or towel

Dance Off the Inches: Dance It Off Ballroom

Focus: Cardio

Why we love it: You'll peel off pounds as you gracefully twirl around your living room with these easy-to-follow routines featuring samba, cha-cha, and jive.

151

The Workouts

Here's how to mix and match these DVDs to meet your fitness goals.

GOAL #1: "I NEED TO START EXERCISING"
If it's been a while since you worked up a sweat, this is the program for you. Starting with a manageable 18 minutes a day, you'll safely build an exercise habit you can stick with. The short bouts of high-energy toning can be broken up throughout the day to fit into even the busiest schedule. And the anyone-can-do-them dance moves will make working out fun (no partner required).

Monday
  DVD: *Total Body Calorie Blast*
  Play: Total Body A (6 minutes), Mind Body A (6 minutes), Quick Abs Blast (6 minutes)
  Total time: 18 minutes

Wednesday
  DVD: *Total Body Calorie Blast*
  Play: Total Body B (6 minutes), Mind Body B (6 minutes), Quick Abs Blast (6 minutes)
  Total time: 18 minutes

Friday
  DVD: *Total Body Calorie Blast*
  Play: Total Body C (6 minutes), Mind Body C (6 minutes), Quick Abs Blast (6 minutes)
  DVD: *Dance It Off Ballroom*
  Play: First week: Step Guide (18 minutes). Subsequent weeks: Samba (10 minutes), Jive (10 minutes)
  Total time: 36 to 38 minutes

Saturday
  DVD: *Dance It Off Ballroom*
  Play: All (42 minutes)
  Total time: 42 minutes

GOAL #2: "I WANT TO FLATTEN MY BELLY"
We've enlisted a three-tiered flab-fighting fix: cardio to melt fat, targeted toning to shrink your waist, and yoga to de-stress.

Monday
  DVD: *Dance It Off Ballroom*
  Play: First week: Step Guide (18 minutes). Subsequent weeks: Samba (10 minutes), Jive (10 minutes)
  DVD: *Quick Tummy Toners*
  Play: Crunch-Free Abs (10 minutes)
  Total time: 28 to 30 minutes

Tuesday
  DVD: *Kick-Start Your Metabolism*
  Play: Fat Blast (15 minutes), Ab Attack (15 minutes)
  DVD: *Quick Tummy Toners*
  Play: Yoga Abs (10 minutes)
  Total time: 40 minutes

Wednesday
  DVD: *Dance It Off Ballroom*
  Play: Cha-Cha (10 minutes), Samba (10 minutes)
  DVD: *Quick Tummy Toners*
  Play: Bikini Belly (10 minutes)
  Total time: 30 minutes

Friday

DVD: *Dance It Off Ballroom*
Play: Samba (10 minutes), Jive (10 minutes)
DVD: *Quick Tummy Toners*
Play: Ab and Waist Definer (10 minutes)
Total time: 30 minutes

Saturday

DVD: *Dance It Off Ballroom*
Play: Cha-Cha (10 minutes), Samba (10 minutes)
DVD: *Quick Tummy Toners*
Play: Yoga Abs (10 minutes), Sporty Abs (10 minutes)
Total time: 40 minutes

Sunday

DVD: *Kick-Start Your Metabolism*
Play: Fat Blast (15 minutes), Ab Attack (15 minutes)
DVD: *Body Sculpt* (15 minutes)
Total time: 45 minutes

GOAL #3: "I NEED TO JUMP-START MY WEIGHT LOSS"

A precise mix of fat-melting cardio and sculpting moves is just the recipe for shedding pounds. This routine obliterates calories with kickboxing and dance, then sculpts metabolism-boosting muscle. Shave 250 calories per day from your diet, and you'll be about a size smaller in 30 days.

■ WEEKS 1 AND 2

Monday

DVD: *Kick-Start Your Metabolism*
Play: Fat Blast (15 minutes), Ab Attack (15 minutes), Body Sculpt (15 minutes)
DVD: *Dance It Off Ballroom*
Play: First week: Step Guide (18 minutes). Second week: Samba (10 minutes), Cha-Cha (10 minutes)
Total time: 63 to 65 minutes

Tuesday

DVD: *Dance It Off Ballroom*
Play: All (42 minutes)
DVD: *Core Fusion Pilates Plus*
Play: Thigh and Gluteus (10 minutes), Flat Back/Round Back (10 minutes)
Total time: 62 minutes

Wednesday

DVD: *Kick-Start Your Metabolism*
Play: Fat Blast (15 minutes), Ab Attack (15 minutes)
DVD: *Core Fusion Pilates Plus*
Play: Upper Body (10 minutes)
Total time: 40 minutes

Thursday

DVD: *Dance It Off Ballroom*
Play: All (42 minutes)
DVD: *Core Fusion Pilates Plus*
Play: Thigh and Gluteus (10 minutes)
Total time: 52 minutes

Saturday
DVD: *Dance It Off Ballroom*
Play: Cha-Cha (10 minutes), Jive (10 minutes)
DVD: *Core Fusion Pilates Plus*
Play: Upper Body (10 minutes), Flat Back/Round Back (10 minutes), Pure Core (10 minutes)
Total time: 50 minutes

Sunday
DVD: *Kick-Start Your Metabolism*
Play: Fat Blast (15 minutes), Ab Attack (15 minutes), Body Sculpt (15 minutes)
Total time: 45 minutes

■ WEEKS 3 AND 4
Monday
DVD: *Dance It Off Ballroom*
Play: All (42 minutes)
DVD: *Kick-Start Your Metabolism*
Play: Ab Attack (15 minutes)
Total time: 57 minutes

Tuesday
DVD: *Kick-Start Your Metabolism*
Play: Fat Blast (15 minutes), Express Kick-Start (10 minutes)
DVD: *Core Fusion Pilates Plus*
Play: Thigh and Gluteus (10 minutes), Flat Back/Round Back (10 minutes), Core Flexibility (10 minutes)
Total time: 55 minutes

Wednesday
DVD: *Dance It Off Ballroom*
Play: All (42 minutes)
DVD: *Core Fusion Pilates Plus*
Play: Upper Body (10 minutes)
Total time: 52 minutes

Thursday
DVD: *Dance It Off Ballroom*
Play: All (42 minutes)
DVD: *Core Fusion Pilates Plus*
Play: Pure Core (10 minutes)
Total time: 52 minutes

Saturday
DVD: *Kick-Start Your Metabolism*
Play: Fat Blast (15 minutes), Body Sculpt (15 minutes)
DVD: *Core Fusion Pilates Plus*
Play: Thigh and Gluteus (10 minutes), Flat Back/Round Back (10 minutes), Upper Body (10 minutes)
Total time: 60 minutes

Sunday
DVD: *Kick-Start Your Metabolism*
Play: All (67 minutes)
Total time: 67 minutes

Get more workouts! Follow your choice of the routines above for 2 weeks. Then you'll be ready to take it to the next level. Get additional weeks at www.prevention.com/dvdworkout.

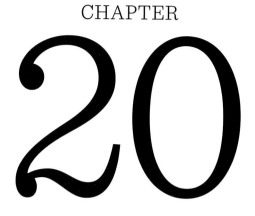

Walk Away from

DIABETES

Flatten your abs, rev your energy, and stabilize your blood sugar with our easy, exclusive routine.

There's no question that walking is great for everyone: It dramatically boosts energy levels, fights fat, and protects the heart. But if you have high blood sugar, or if you have been diagnosed with prediabetes or diabetes, walking can literally be a lifesaver.

"Walking is one of the best types of 'medicine' we have to help prevent diabetes or reduce its severity and potential complications—such as heart attack and stroke—if you already have it," says JoAnn E. Manson, MD, DrPH, chief of the division of preventive medicine at Brigham and Women's Hospital in Boston and a professor of medicine at Harvard Medical School.

Women who did at least 30 minutes daily of moderate physical activity, such as brisk walking, slashed their risk of diabetes by 30 percent, the Harvard Nurses' Health Study found. Even a single 90-minute session of aerobic exercise improved blood sugar control in at-risk women, according to research at the University of Michigan.

Walking also shrinks dangerous abdominal fat. Excess fat around your abdomen causes inflammation in cells, making them even more resistant to insulin, which increases your odds of developing the disease. A Canadian study found that women who walked briskly for about an hour a day decreased their belly fat by 20 percent after 14 weeks—without changing their eating habits.

The best medicine of all is likely combining walking and toning exercises.

"Together, the two build lean muscle and help reduce body fat—a combination

Workout at a Glance

What you'll need: Supportive athletic shoes, watch with timer, mat

What you'll do: Six workouts a week: Fat-Torch Walk (2 days a week), a steady-paced workout to burn flab

Calorie-Scorch Walk (2 days a week), short intervals of fast walking to rev up your metabolism so you burn more calories all day long

Belly Blast Routine (2 days a week), a 15-minute toning routine designed to firm your core—abs, lower back, and butt. Studies suggest that adding strength training to your workouts improves blood sugar more than doing just cardio.

For faster results: Check out www.prevention.com/dtour for tips, meals, and success stories.

Get Started

Day	Activity
1	Fat-Torch Walk* (20 min)
2	Belly Blast Routine (15 min)
3	Calorie-Scorch Walk* (15 min)
4	Rest
5	Fat-Torch Walk (20 min)
6	Belly Blast Routine (15 min)
7	Calorie-Scorch Walk (15 min)

that can dramatically improve blood sugar," says Francine R. Kaufman, MD, head of the Center for Endocrinology, Diabetes, and Metabolism at Childrens Hospital Los Angeles.

Here's a plan so you can get started today. In just 2 weeks, you could lose a few pounds, shrink your waistline, and improve your blood sugar levels.

THE WALKS

Fat-Torch Walk

Time	Activity	Speed	Intensity
0:00	Warmup	3–3.5 mph	Light: You can sing.
3:00	Cardio walk	3.5–4 mph	Moderate: You can chat with a friend.
18:00	Cooldown	3–3.5 mph	
20:00	Finish		

Note: Each week, increase the cardio walk portion by 5 minutes; build up to a 60-minute workout.

Calorie-Scorch Walk

Time	Activity	Speed	Intensity
0:00	Warmup	3–3.5 mph	Light: You can sing.
3:00	Cardio walk	3.5–4 mph	Moderate: You can chat with a friend.
4:00	Speed walk	4-plus mph	Vigorous: You can barely talk.
4:30	Repeat 1-min cardio walk and 30-sec speed walk intervals 5 more times.		
12:00	Cardio walk		
13:00	Cooldown	3–3.5 mph	

THE BELLY BLAST ROUTINE

Do this workout twice a week. It's a 15-minute routine that's designed to firm your core. Studies suggest that adding strength training to your workouts improves blood sugar more than cardio alone can.

Crisscross

> Lie on your back with your feet off the floor, your knees at 90 degrees, and your hands behind your head. (A) Contract your abs, press your lower back toward the floor, and curl your head and neck off the floor. (B) Inhale and extend your left leg while drawing your right knee toward your chest. At the same time, twist to bring your left elbow toward your right knee. Exhale and twist to the left, switching legs. That's 1 rep; do 6.

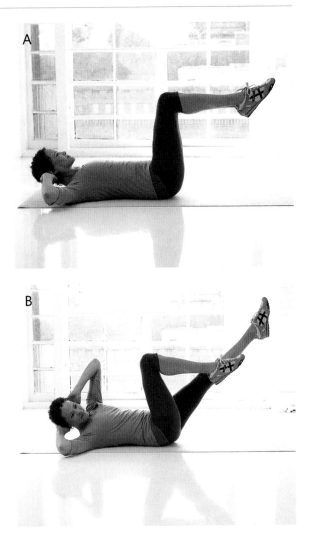

Leg Circle

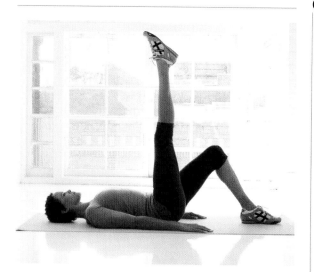

> Lie on your back with your left foot flat on the floor, your right leg extended toward the ceiling, your toes pointed, and your arms at your sides. Hold for 10 to 60 seconds. Then, keeping your abs tight, rotate your right leg from the hip in small circles. Inhale as you begin the circle; exhale as you finish. Do 6 circles; repeat in the opposite direction. Switch legs. (For a challenge, straighten your left leg.)

CONVENIENT CARRYALLS

Hidden pockets in this genius walking gear make toting your stuff a breeze—so you can focus on your workout.

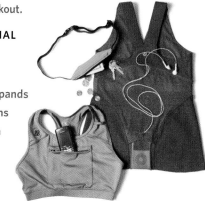

SPIBELT PERSONAL ITEM BELT

This waist pack's stretchy fabric expands to hold larger items (such as a camera for scenic hikes), and it shrinks when all you have is a key and an ID. The elastic band lies comfortably snug, so it won't ride up (www.spibelt.com).

GRACIE'S GEAR SHORT TOP

If you've ever stashed cash in your sports bra, this top is for you: A zippered pouch at the bust has three built-in compartments that hold items separately to minimize movement and bulk (www.graciesgear andtraining.com).

LULULEMON ATHLETIC DEEP V TANK

A lower back pocket in this full-coverage tank holds your iPod securely, while a special cord lacing system prevents tangles. Load your favorite playlist ahead of time to put your music on autopilot (www.lululemon. com for stores).

Get more smart pocket gear at www.prevention. com/handsfree.

Leg Kick

> Lie on your right side, propped on your right elbow and forearm, your torso lifted off the floor, your legs stacked and in line with your body, and your left hand in front for balance.
> (A) Exhale and slowly swing your left leg forward as far as it's comfortable. Hold and pulse, moving your left foot forward and back a few inches, for 2 counts.
> (B) Inhale and swing your leg back, past the right one. Do 6 times without lowering your leg. Switch sides. (For an easier option, extend your right arm on the floor and rest your head on that arm.)

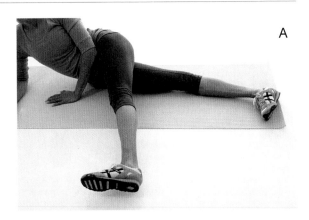

A

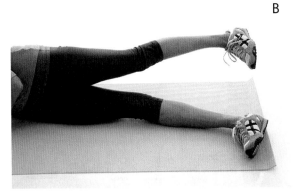

B

Fight Fat
OVER 40

Staying slim and strong for life is all about metabolism. Our new plan burns an extra 500 calories a day so **you can double your weight loss each month.**

I s your wardrobe suddenly shrinking? If you're over 40, it's probably not your clothing or an overactive dryer but, rather, an underactive metabolism that's to blame. It can dip by as much as 200 calories per day from your midtwenties to your midfifties, which is enough to pack on nearly an extra 30 pounds in that time. And that old weight loss strategy of crash dieting will just make it worse. What you need is a smarter approach to losing fat while building muscle, which powers your calorie burn and is key to reversing a slow metabolism.

We combed through the very latest research and talked to top experts to create our Ultimate Over-40 Fat-Fighting Workout. It's a unique blend of calorie-blasting cardio, supercharged strength training, and lifestyle tips that will help you burn calories at a higher rate (even while you're sleeping) than you did in your twenties—up to an extra 500 calories a day! That's enough for you to double your weight loss and drop a size this month. Soon your only wardrobe worry will be buying smaller sizes!

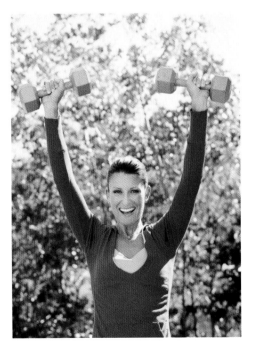

Fire Up Your Metabolism: Cardio Tips

The latest research shows that simple changes to your cardio workouts can boost calorie burn by 25 to 50 percent. Our routines include the following four rules to guarantee a high calorie burn.

Always warm up: It raises your core body temperature and increases the activity of fat-burning enzymes, explains exercise physiologist Chip Harrison, director of strength and fitness at Pennsylvania State University and coauthor of *The Female Athlete*. For each degree your body temp goes up, the metabolic rate inside your cells increases by about 13 percent. Warm up by doing your activity at an easy to moderate intensity for at least 5 minutes to gradually raise your heart rate, send blood to your working muscles, ramp up your respiration, and get the maximum boost in calorie burn.

Three More Ways to Fight Fat after 40

Pump up your natural calorie burn with the following simple tips.

Work out with music: It can help you go up to 20 percent longer to burn more calories, finds a study from West London's Brunel University. Music blocks fatigue, produces feelings of vigor, and helps you keep pace by synchronizing your movements, according to study author Costas Karageorghis, PhD. For workouts set to music, go to www.prevention.com/podcasts.

Take it outside: Research finds that exercisers burn 10 percent more calories when they walk or run outdoors than they do on a treadmill at the same speed. "You use more energy to propel yourself over the ground," explains fitness expert Jay Blahnik, author of *Full-Body Flexibility*, "and pushing a little against the wind or other elements burns more calories, too."

Move more all day: You can burn up to 350 extra calories daily—enough to shed more than 35 pounds a year—simply by pacing while you talk on the phone, getting up to talk to someone rather than e-mailing a few times a day, and walking rather than driving for short errands, advises James A. Levine, MD, PhD, of the Mayo Clinic and author of *Move a Little, Lose a Lot*.

Do at least 12 minutes: Any amount of cardio will burn calories, but to really fight off post-40 pounds, you need at least 12 minutes (beyond a warmup) of continuously moderate to high-intensity activity (where you're breathing somewhat hard) most days of the week. That's the amount necessary to "create a training effect, which improves your body's ability to use oxygen and generate more fat-burning enzymes, such as lipase, so you can blast more flab during exercise and other activities all day," says Harrison.

Commit to intervals: Studies show that workouts with bursts of high-intensity activity can boost your calorie burn more than steady-paced training can. "Interval training increases the mitochondrial activity in the muscle, which is a scientific way of saying it increases your cells' fat-burning capacity," says exercise physiologist Jason Talanian, PhD, formerly of the University of Guelph in Ontario.

Because intervals are harder than one-speed workouts, it takes more time for your body to return to normal afterward, so your calorie burn stays elevated longer. In a College of New Jersey study of 48 men and women, researchers found that those who rode stationary bikes at varying intensities, such as pedaling just a little harder for 5 minutes and then a little easier for 5 minutes over a half-hour workout, burned about 15 percent more calories for about 30 minutes after their sessions than did their peers who stuck to one moderate pace the entire time.

Devote 1 hour once a week: Going longer gives you a big metabolic boost because your body has to reach into its reserves and expend a lot of energy replenishing its fuel stores and repairing broken-down muscle fibers when you're finished. In one small study, researchers at the University of Victoria in British Columbia found that exercisers who chugged along

YOUR 7-DAY SAMPLE SCHEDULE

Here's 1 week of workouts to get you into the swing of things.

Monday: Steady Cardio and Strength
(40 min total)

Tuesday: Interval Fat Blast
(30 min total)

Wednesday: Steady Cardio and Strength
(40 min total)

Thursday: Interval Fat Blast
(30 min total)

Friday: Steady Cardio and Strength
(40 min total)

Saturday: Interval Fat Blast
(30 min total)

Sunday: Endurance Builder
(60 min total).

for 60 minutes burned nearly five times as many calories postworkout as those who did only 30 minutes of activity.

Fire Up Your Metabolism: Strength Tips

Strength training is essential. Lean muscle tissue burns about three times as many calories as fat and is the power behind your metabolism. But how you do it can speed your calorie burn by up to an extra 25 percent.

Break up your sets: Instead of performing 2 or 3 sets of a single exercise before moving to the next one, do a circuit: Complete just 1 set and then immediately move to the next exercise, repeating the circuit two or three times. When researchers had 10 men do either standard strength training (3 sets of six exercises with 2 minutes of rest in between) or circuit training (moving through a series of six exercises three times, with 30 seconds of rest in between), the circuit trainers burned nearly twice as many calories postworkout as the standard-style lifters.

"Because your heart rate stays elevated longer after circuit training, you continue burning fat as though you were still exercising," says researcher Anthony Caterisano, PhD, of Furman University in Greenville, South Carolina.

Grab the heavy dumbbells: Even when exercisers lifted identical volumes (such as 10 pounds 10 times or 20 pounds

5 times), those using the heavier dumb-bells burned about 25 percent more calories when they were finished.

"Heavy weights create more protein breakdown in the muscle, so your body has to use more energy to repair and recover. That's how lean muscle tissue is built," says Dr. Caterisano.

And the boost can last even longer. Researchers at Washington University in St. Louis School of Medicine found that working out with heavy weights even for as few as 3 to 6 reps increased exercisers' sleeping metabolic rate—the number of calories burned overnight—by nearly 8 percent. That's enough to

30-Minute Interval Fat Blast

This workout is the first portion of our three-part metabolism-boosting cardio plan. Choose your favorite form of aerobic exercise, such as walking, cycling, or swimming. To reap the full benefits, just be sure to pay attention to the changes in workout intensity.

Time	Activity	Intensity*
0:00	Warmup	3, working up to 6 (rhythmic breathing; can speak easily)
5:00	Brisk pace	7–8 (harder breathing; can speak in very short sentences only)
8:00	Moderate pace	5–6 (breathing somewhat hard; can speak in full sentences)
10:00	Fast pace	9 (no speaking; just hard but controlled breathing)
12:00	Do 2-min moderate and 2-min fast intervals 3 more times.	
24:00	Moderate pace	5–6
26:00	Brisk pace	7–8
28:00	Cooldown	Work down to a 3
30:00	Finished	

*Based on a 1-to-10 scale, with 1 being as easy as lounging on the couch and 10 as hard as sprinting to catch a bus as it pulls away.

lose about 5 pounds in a year, even if you did nothing else.

Program at a Glance

FIRE UP METABOLISM: CARDIO

You'll walk or do aerobic exercise such as jogging, swimming, or cycling every day, alternating three different routines to maximize fat burn.

Three times a week: 30-Minute Interval Fat Blast (page 165). Alternate 2-minute bursts of high-intensity activity with 2-minute bouts of moderate intensity to boost calorie burn during and after exercise.

Three times a week: 20-Minute Steady Cardio. After a 5-minute warmup, exercise at a pace that keeps your heart rate in an aerobic zone (where you're breathing somewhat hard) for 12 minutes, then slow your pace for 3 minutes to cool down. You'll burn extra calories while allowing your body to recover from the more intense interval days.

Quick Tip

Swing your arms. Bend your elbows 90 degrees and pump your arms as you walk. This action automatically speeds up your pace, and it also helps you burn up to 15 percent more calories every time you work out.

One time a week: 60-Minute Endurance Builder. Warm up for 5 minutes, then increase to a moderate intensity for the rest of the workout. Going longer will crank up your postexercise calorie burn and increase stamina so all your workouts feel easier.

FIRE UP METABOLISM: STRENGTH

Three times a week: On days you do the Steady Cardio workout, you'll also do our 20-minute high-energy dumbbell routine, the Strength Circuit, to build more metabolism-stoking muscle and firm up all over.

The Strength Circuit

What to do: Complete the circuit three times, moving immediately from one exercise to the next with minimal to no rest between moves. The first time through, do 8 to 12 reps of each move with a lighter weight as a warmup. For the second and third sets, use an amount that you're able to lift no more than 8 to 10 times.

How often: 3 nonconsecutive days a week, preferably when you do the Steady Cardio workouts

What you'll need: 1 pair of light weights (5 to 10 pounds), 1 set of heavier dumbbells (10 to 15 pounds; for some exercises, you may need even heavier weights), stability ball (optional)

The expert: Valerie Waters, a certified trainer in Brentwood, California, and author of *Red Carpet Ready*, designed this workout.

THE STRENGTH CIRCUIT

Step Squat

Firms glutes and thighs

> Hold the dumbbells at your sides, palms in, and stand with a low step about 2 feet behind you. Extend your left leg behind you and place the top of your foot on the step. Bend your right leg and lower hips, keeping your front knee behind your toes, until your right thigh is about parallel to the floor. Return to the start position. Complete a full set, then switch sides.

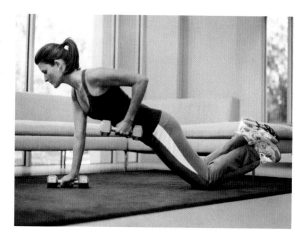

Plank Row

Firms shoulders, back, and abs

> Hold a dumbbell in each hand and assume a modified pushup position (your hands beneath your shoulders, knees on the floor, ankles crossed in the air). Keeping your torso steady, bend your left elbow and pull the dumbbell up toward your rib cage. Lower and repeat with the right arm. Alternate arms for a full set. For a challenge, perform the move with your legs extended, balancing on your toes.

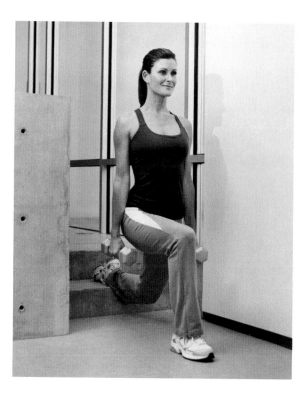

THE STRENGTH CIRCUIT (CONT.)

Wall-Sit Arm Curl

Firms arms, glutes, and thighs

> Hold a dumbbell in each hand, palms facing forward, and stand with your back against the wall. Slide down the wall until your legs are bent 90 degrees. Bend your elbows and lift the weights toward your shoulders, then lower. Complete a full set of arm curls before returning to the standing position.

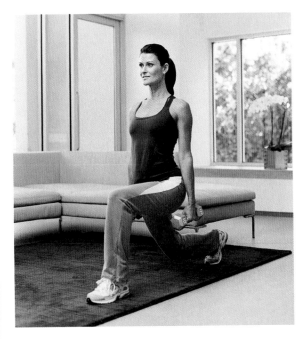

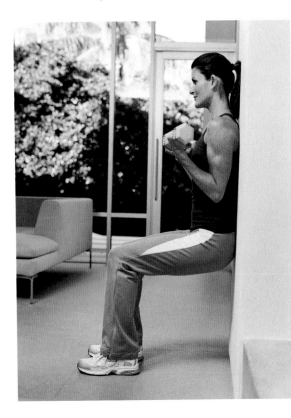

Pendulum Lunge

Firms glutes and thighs

> Hold the dumbbells at your sides, palms in, and stand with your feet close together. Take a giant step back with your right leg, bend your knees, and lower until your left thigh is parallel to the floor, keeping your front knee behind your toes (as shown). Press into your left foot to stand back up and bring your right leg forward, stepping into a front lunge. Continue stepping back and front for a full set with your right leg, then repeat with the left.

Ball Chest Press

Firms shoulders, chest, arms, and glutes

› Holding the dumbbells, lie on a stability
ball (your head, shoulders, and upper
back supported) so that your body forms a
straight line (like a tabletop) from your
head to your knees. Position the weights
at chest height, your elbows pointing to
your sides, and your palms facing your
toes). Keeping your torso steady,
straighten your arms and press the
weights toward the ceiling. Lower
weights. Repeat for a full set. No stability
ball? Perform the move off the edge of a
bed, sofa, or deep-seated chair.

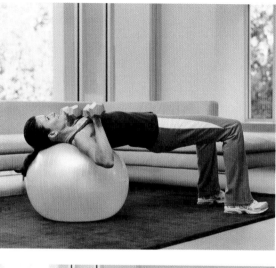

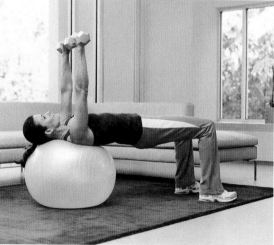

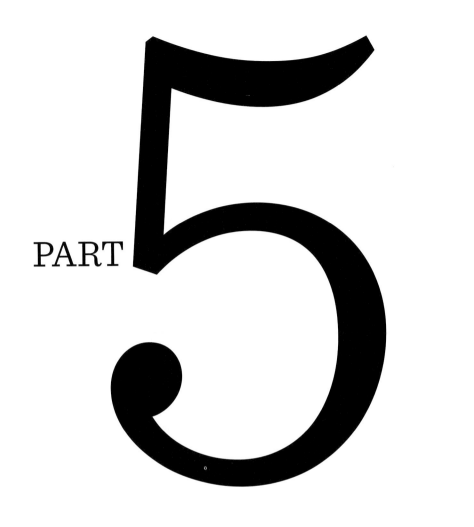

5

MIND

MATTERS

connection becomes even more important—and clear.

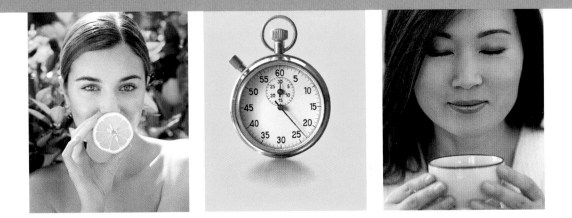

MIND-BODY
Medical Breakthroughs

Just as how your body feels affects your mental state, the way your mind feels affects your body. Stress, for example, can alter your blood sugar. If you're under stress, you might not eat as well, exercise, or limit drinking, all of which can raise blood glucose. On the other hand, **if you have the right mental attitude, you're more likely to take better care of yourself.**

DON'T WORRY YOURSELF INTO DIABETES

Stress doesn't do a body good, especially not a body with diabetes. The fight-or-flight response causes a surge in stress hormones, which in turn prompts your liver to make a lot of stored energy (sugar and fat) available to cells so that they have the necessary fuel to power the body to react. (So you could have outrun that woolly mammoth that was chasing you!) In a person without diabetes, the healthy pancreas recognizes this rise in blood sugar and secretes the hormone insulin in response.

But this isn't what happens if you have diabetes. Either the pancreas is unable to secrete insulin, or cells are unable to respond to the hormone. The result is the same: Blood sugar goes up and stays up.

Researchers who study diabetes continue to ponder whether stress could be a precursor to the disease. Based on the current state of the science, the answer appears to be yes. One study of 677 Israeli workers found that the folks with job burnout were almost twice as likely to develop type 2 diabetes, even when the scientists accounted for factors such as age, sex, activity level, and obesity.

In an earlier study, researchers at the University of Washington compared 47 people who were the caregivers for spouses with Alzheimer's disease, which certainly can be stressful, with 77 who were not. Levels of cortisol, glucose, and insulin all turned out to be higher in the caregivers than in the noncaregivers.

LAUGH IT UP

Looking for an excuse to catch a comedy show or spend time with a funny friend? Look no further.

In a small study, researchers in Japan examined 19 people with diabetes. The scientists were able to link laughter to lower blood sugar after a meal. They think that laughter affects the neuroendocrine system, which monitors the body's blood sugar levels. And that's no laughing matter.

BE HAPPY, BE HEALTHY

Staying happy can have as powerful an impact on your physical health as avoiding cigarettes does, according to Dutch social scientist Ruut Veenhoven, PhD. He analyzed 30 past studies and found that happiness helps bolster the immune system and prevents healthy people from falling ill, tacking on on extra years of life as a result. That's a lot to be happy about.

SPEND HAPPY

To get more happiness for your dollar, splurge on experiences instead of stuff. Psychologist Miriam Tatzel, PhD, of Empire State College, State University of New York, in Saratoga Springs, surveyed 329 shoppers and found that "experiencers"—consumers who are easygoing about spending on a great meal out or a concert, for example—are happier than those who

Additional times per year that "very happy" people—compared with unhappy people—visit with neighbors, according to *Social Indicators Research*, 2008:

7

lavish their money on material goods such as clothes or jewelry. A bonus: Experiences allow you to spend high-quality time with family and friends; a new pair of shoes is a solo endeavor.

FEEL BETTER—FAST

For an instant mood lift, sit or stand up straighter. When Ohio State University researchers asked study participants to rate their skills related to job opportunities, they found that those who completed the task with proper posture were more secure in their abilities than those who were slumped over.

"People feel confident when they're sitting upright, and they can attribute that confidence to their present thoughts," says study author and psychologist Richard E. Petty, PhD.

BOOST YOUR MOOD

Turn your thoughts into a race; it can lift the blues in minutes, advises Princeton University psychologist Emily Pronin, PhD. For example, if your mother-in-law is driving you crazy, allow yourself 30 seconds to make a list of all the ways she's been helpful to you in the past. You'll feel better fast. (If nothing nice comes to mind, quickly jot down other ways that she bugs you; speed-thinking negative thoughts can also improve your mood, Dr. Pronin found.) Researchers say that rapid thinking may release feel-good neurotransmitters, or it could just be a helpful distraction.

The percentage of adults who believe that their stress levels have increased over the previous year, according to an American Psychological Association Stress in America Survey:

47

COVET THY NEIGHBOR'S HAPPINESS

Socializing with a cheerful person in your neighborhood increases the likelihood that you'll be happy, too—much more so, in fact, than spending time with an upbeat sibling, according to a new study. How often you get together matters most, according to the researchers: People who live within half a mile of a buoyant buddy increase their odds of being happy by 42 percent. If the friend lives farther away (within a 2-mile radius), the chances drop to 22 percent—probably because of fewer get-togethers.

SPOT SILENT STRESS SIGNALS

The occasional manic Monday is a fact of modern life, but if you're under chronic stress—suffering a daily assault of stress hormones from a demanding job or a personal life in turmoil—symptoms may be subtler, says Stevan E. Hobfoll, PhD, chair of the department of behavioral sciences at Rush University Medical Center. If you experience any of the signs below, take some time out every day, he says—whether it's to go for a walk or simply turn off your phone.

Weekend headaches: A sudden drop in stress can prompt migraines, says Todd Schwedt, MD, director of the Washington University Headache Center. Stick closely to your weekday sleeping and eating schedule to minimize other triggers.

Awful menstrual cramps: The most stressed women are more than twice as likely to get painful cramps as those who are less tense, found a Harvard School of Public Health study. Researchers blame a stress-induced imbalance of hormones. Exercise can soothe cramps and stress by decreasing sympathetic nervous system activity.

An achy mouth: A sore jaw may be a sign of teeth grinding, which can be worsened by stress, says Matthew Messina, DDS, a consumer advisor to the American Dental Association. Ask your dentist about a nighttime mouth guard. Up to 70 percent of people who use one reduce grinding or stop it altogether.

Odd dreams: Dreams usually get progressively more positive as you sleep, so you wake up happier than you were before bed, says Rosalind Cartwright, PhD, an emeritus professor of psychology at Rush University Medical Center. When stressed, you wake up more often, disrupting this process and allowing unpleasant imagery all night. Good sleep habits can help prevent this; aim for 7 to 8 hours a night, and avoid caffeine and alcohol close to bedtime.

▤ GET INSTANT CALM AT WORK

Frazzled on the job but too busy to do anything about it? Just four "minirelaxation" sessions ($1\frac{1}{2}$ to 2 minutes) over the course of the day reduced work-related stress as effectively as 15-minute blocks of progressive muscle relaxation, according to a University of Connecticut study. During the minisessions, participants were simply instructed to relax; breathe slowly and deeply; and imagine a peaceful, serene place. The tests also found that subjects were more willing to stick with minirelaxation in the future because it takes up so little time.

▤ SNIFF YOUR WAY CALM

Japanese researchers recently found that when animals under stress were exposed to the compound linalool—a fragrant substance found in lemons as well as in mango, lavender, basil, and some teas—they experienced lower levels of inflammatory chemicals in their blood, compared with another group that did not smell the linalool. Inhaling the scent also reduced the activity of more than 100 genes that are activated during stressful situations.

▤ WALK FOR HAPPIER HORMONES

Exercise might be key to a sunny outlook through perimenopause and beyond, a new study has found. Inactive women ages 42 to 58 who did about 3 hours of moderate activity (such as walking) per week felt happier and more confident about their bodies over a 2-year period, and they also noticed a drop in hot flashes and night sweats. One explanation might be that exercise elevates levels of endorphins that foster feelings of well-being, help you relax, and affect your ability to regulate body temp.

The minutes of exercise a day that can boost your mood and body confidence, according to *Menopause: The Journal of the North American Menopause Society:*

25

▦ GO NATURAL

Working up a sweat may be the easiest, most effective way to stay calm without pills, according to a new study. Arizona State University researchers analyzed a host of strategies, including meditation, yoga, stretching, and talk therapy; only prescription meds reduced anxiety better than moderate to vigorous exercise. The scientists found that burning about 850 calories a week—a 30-minute brisk walk or 15-minute jog daily, on average—is an optimal anxiety-easing goal for many.

▦ HELP OTHERS TO HELP YOURSELF

More than 60 percent of centenarians say that they help others as a way to relieve stress, compared with 44 percent of college seniors, found a recent survey that compared the lifestyle habits of the two groups. College students were more apt to relax by setting aside "me time" than the centenarian group was.

Beat Your Stress
HORMONES

Managing cortisol can help you **think faster, slim down, and even avoid a cold.**

Poor cortisol—it means well but just doesn't know when to quit. Produced by your adrenal glands, this "stress hormone" helps regulate blood pressure and the immune system during a sudden crisis, whether a physical attack or an emotional setback. This helps you tap into your energy reserves and increases your ability to fight off infection.

Trouble is, relentless stress can keep this survival mechanism revving in high gear, subverting the hormone's good intentions. Chronically high cortisol levels can cause blood sugar abnormalities, sleep problems, a depressed immune response, and even abdominal weight gain.

"When cortisol spikes, it tells the body to eat something with a lot of calories—a great survival tactic if you need energy to flee a predator, but not if you're fretting over how to pay bills," says nutritional biochemist Shawn M. Talbott, PhD, author of *The Cortisol Connection.*

Fortunately, an antidote to the body's fight-or-flight mode has evolved: the relaxation response. Here are eight surprising ways to invoke it—and, in some cases, cut your cortisol levels almost in half.

Say "Om"

Cut cortisol by 20 percent.

Subjects who practiced Buddhist meditation significantly decreased both their cortisol levels and blood pressure in a 6-week Thai study. Similarly, participants who meditated daily for 4 months

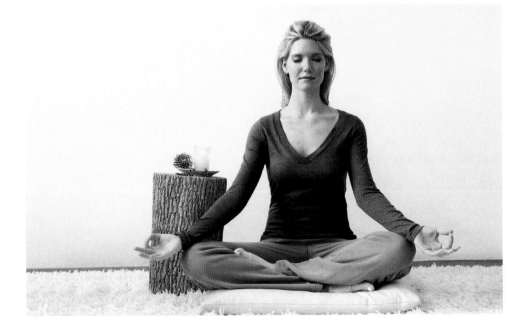

decreased their levels of the hormone by an average of 20 percent in a study at Maharishi University, while levels in the nonmeditating control group actually went up slightly. Visit www.prevention.com/meditate to learn about meditation's other stress-relieving benefits.

Make a Great iPod Mix

Cut cortisol by 66 percent.

Music can have a calming effect on the brain, especially while you're facing down a major stressor. When doctors at Japan's Osaka Medical Center played tunes for a group of patients undergoing colonoscopies, the patients' cortisol levels rose less than those of others who underwent the same procedure in a quiet room. Even if an invasive gastrointestinal exam isn't in your immediate future, you can forestall cortisol spikes in other stressful situations—when hosting dinner for your in-laws, for instance—by queuing up background music. And to wind down faster at bedtime, listen to something soothing instead of watching TV.

Hit the Sack Early— Or Take a Nap

Cut cortisol by 50 percent.

What's the difference between getting 6 hours of sleep and the suggested 8?

"Fifty percent more cortisol in the bloodstream," Dr. Talbott says.

When a group of pilots slept 6 hours or

The Good Side of Stress

Under the right circumstances, a little bit of cortisol can be helpful. Here are a few examples.

Boost sex drive: Women who took 20 sniffs of a bottle containing a component of male sweat, a reported pheromone, experienced surges in mood, sexual arousal, and cortisol levels within 15 minutes, found a study from the University of California, Berkeley.

Ease pain: Patients suffering from chronic fatigue syndrome or fibromyalgia who took customized cortisol doses improved symptoms by 75 percent. Researchers speculate that cortisol may help kick certain hormone-producing systems back into high gear.

Improve memory: A study of 90 men done by the University of Wisconsin–Madison found that moderate levels of cortisol translated into better performance on memory tests, although very high levels—"from too much stress"—reduced the effect (meaning poorer recall).

less for 7 nights while on duty, their cortisol levels increased significantly and stayed elevated for 2 days, found a study at Germany's Institute of Aerospace Medicine. Getting the recommended 8 hours of nightly shut-eye allows your body enough time to recover from the day's stresses, according to Dr. Talbott. When you fall short of the mark, take a nap the next day. Pennsylvania State University researchers found that a midday snooze cut cortisol levels in subjects who'd lost sleep the previous night.

Sip Some Black Tea

Cut cortisol by 47 percent.

The "cup that cheers" has deep associations with comfort and calm; just think of how the English revere their late-afternoon teatime. As it turns out, science confirms the connection: When volunteers at University College London were given a stressful task, those who regularly drank black tea experienced a 47 percent drop in their cortisol levels within an hour of completing the assign-

THE STRESS-DIABETES CONNECTION

Deadlines, bills, commitments . . . Chronic stress is practically a lifestyle for many Americans.

But all that stress has a dramatic impact on blood sugar levels. It prompts your liver to make a lot of sugar and fat available to your cells so that you have the energy to react to whatever's causing your stress. If your pancreas is healthy, it could recognize this increase in blood sugar and secrete insulin in response. The pancreas of a person with diabetes, however, isn't able to do this, so her blood sugar goes up and stays up.

To compound things, chronic stress also contributes to weight gain. This is partly because all that cortisol coursing through your bloodstream triggers cravings for high-fat, high-sugar comfort foods. (Yes, I would like fries with that!) This might help explain why many of us turn to food when we're stressed-out and why we're likely to choose a brownie rather than a nice bowl of steamed broccoli. Plus, if you're stressed, it's an easy excuse to trade your workout time for couch time.

The continual flood of cortisol that occurs with chronic stress contributes to weight gain in another way: by instructing the body to store fat around the belly. It's nature's way of ensuring that you have adequate energy reserves to survive a catastrophic event like, say, a famine.

The good news is that if you're able to control stress, it will help you lower your blood sugar and control your diabetes. In a landmark study conducted at Duke University, 108 people with diabetes attended five diabetes education sessions with or without stress-

ment, while others who drank fake tea had only a 27 percent drop. Study author Andrew Steptoe, PhD, suspects that naturally occurring chemicals such as polyphenols and flavonoids might be responsible for tea's calming effects.

Hang Out with a Funny Friend

Cut cortisol by 39 percent.

The pal who keeps you in stitches can do more than distract you from your problems. Her very presence might help temper your hormonal stress response. Simply anticipating laughter is enough to reduce cortisol levels by nearly half, according to researchers at Loma Linda University.

If your favorite Tina Fey clone can't meet for coffee, you might be able to achieve the same stress-melting effect by popping in a DVD of *The Office* or *Groundhog Day*.

Schedule a Massage

Cut cortisol by 31 percent.

A little pampering can rub your stress

management training, which included a technique called progressive muscle relaxation. After a year, one-third of the patients in the stress-management group had improved their blood sugar levels enough to lower their risk of the most serious diabetes complications, such as heart disease, kidney failure, nerve damage, and vision problems.

More recent studies of a relaxation technique known as mindfulness suggest similar results. Mindfulness essentially means living in the moment. To do it, all you have to do is focus on the here and now instead of dwelling on the past or worrying about the future.

In 1978, pioneering mind-body researcher Jon Kabat-Zinn, PhD, launched the mindfulness-based stress reduction (MBSR) program at the stress-reduction clinic he founded at the University of Massachusetts Medical School.

Researchers in Philadelphia decided to investigate whether MBSR could help people with diabetes manage their blood sugar. For a small 2007 pilot study, they recruited 11 men and women with diabetes to follow the program. The group learned a range of mindfulness meditation techniques, such as awareness of breathing and how to walk, eat, and communicate in mindful ways. They practiced these techniques on their own for at least 20 minutes 6 days a week. After 8 weeks all of the participants showed, on average, a 0.48 percent reduction in their A1C levels (a measure of blood sugar). As a bonus, their self-reported symptoms of depression, anxiety, and stress declined by 43 percent, 37 percent, and 35 percent, respectively.

The present truly is a present.

levels the right way. After several weeks of massage therapy, subjects' cortisol levels decreased, on average, by nearly one-third, according to studies at the University of Miami Miller School of Medicine and elsewhere. In addition to keeping cortisol under control, massage sessions reduce stress by promoting production of dopamine and serotonin, the same feel-good hormones released when we socialize with pals or do something fun.

Do Something Spiritual

Cut cortisol by 25 percent.

Religious ritual fortifies many people against everyday pressures, and it can also lower cortisol secretion, report University of Mississippi researchers. Churchgoing study subjects had lower levels of the stress hormone, on average, than those who did not attend services at all.

If organized religion isn't of interest to you, try developing your spiritual side by taking a walk in nature's "cathedral"—in the woods or along a beach—or volunteering for a charity.

Chew a Piece of Gum

Cut cortisol by 12 to 16 percent.

Next time you feel frazzled, try popping a stick of gum into your mouth to instantly defuse tension, suggest new findings from Northumbria University in the United Kingdom. While under moderate stress, gum chewers had salivary cortisol levels that were 12 percent lower than nonchewers' and also reported greater alertness than their gum-deprived counterparts. One possible mechanism: In past experiments, chewing gum increased blood flow and neural activity in select brain regions.

23

Use Your Willpower

WISELY

New research shows that **you have a finite store of this valuable cognitive currency, and it's actually affected by your blood sugar.** Here's how to spend it the smart way.

Ever heard a doughnut cry out your name? Many people see a sugary snack and want it so badly they can taste it—and then they do. What happened to their willpower?

Many of us struggle with that vexing challenge—whether it's sticking to a new diet or resisting a shopping spree. Why is our self-control so strong on some days and so weak on others?

Contrary to popular belief, willpower is not dependent on psychological strength alone. Physiological factors, such as blood sugar, brain chemistry, and hormones, also influence—and can undermine—our powers of self-restraint. The good news: "Once you understand the forces that weaken your self-control, you can do a lot to strengthen it," says Kathleen D. Vohs, PhD, an associate professor of consumer psychology at the Carlson School of Management in Min-

neapolis. Here's how to reinforce your willpower so it's ready when you need it.

Keep Blood Sugar Steady

Even a small blood sugar dip, which occurs after you've skipped a meal, can impair the areas that oversee planning and self-restraint. Ironically, research shows that exerting your willpower decreases glucose even more. So if you skip lunch and spend the afternoon fighting the desire to dip into a co-worker's candy jar, you could set yourself up for an evening binge.

Tip: Eat small meals that contain both complex carbohydrates and protein

Surprise Craving Fighters

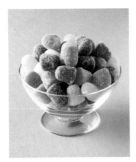

Need a new game plan to outsmart food cravings? Follow the opposite of your instincts, suggest American, Belgian, and Hong Kong researchers in numerous studies.

First, rather than repress memories of other times you succumbed to the tempting food, recall a prior lapse in willpower; this can make it easier for you to resist, researchers say.

Second, don't banish enticing foods; leaving tempting treats like candy in plain view may actually increase willpower and self-control over time.

throughout the day, including breakfast. Keep protein-packed energy bars—with at least 5 grams of protein—in your bag so you never have to skip a meal. By stabilizing blood sugar, you'll be better able to resist overeating—and other impulsive activities—later.

Budget Your Resolve

Each of us has a limited amount of self-control, which means if you try to exert it in too many areas at once, you'll rapidly deplete your supply. A study from Case Western Reserve University illustrates the point.

Researchers placed freshly baked chocolate chip cookies before two groups of participants, instructing one group to eat two or three and the other to eat radishes (while watching the others partake). Then everyone was asked to try to solve an impossible puzzle. Participants who had to resist the treats gave up on the problem twice as fast as those who were allowed to indulge.

"Willpower is like gas in your car," says Dr. Vohs. "When you resist something tempting, you use some up. The more you resist, the emptier your tank gets, until you run out of gas."

Tip: Concentrate your willpower where you need it most. Don't try to cut down on your computer chat time and lose weight at the same time. (And if you've spent the whole day fighting the urge to tell off a difficult colleague, don't go shopping after work. Dr. Vohs found that people were willing to purchase more when their willpower had been drained by a previous unrelated exercise in self-control.)

Don't Overdiet

Eating too little depletes glucose, and it also curtails the production of leptin, which is a hormone made by fat cells that helps regulate appetite.

"Within a few days of starting to diet, your leptin levels can drop by half," explains Neal D. Barnard, MD, author of *Breaking the Food Seduction.* "Plummeting levels can increase appetite and bring on a binge."

Tip: Follow "the rule of 10": Multiply your target weight by 10, and never eat fewer calories than that daily total. And be sure to exercise 30 to 40 minutes each day. (A walk is fine.) Daily activity also maintains healthy levels of leptin, research shows.

Don't Skimp on Sleep

Research indicates that getting less than 6 hours of snooze time decreases your decision-making ability and leads to what Dr. Vohs calls failures of self-control as the day wears on. One mechanism in play: ghrelin, which is a hormone that triggers hunger. One study of healthy adults found that after they got

79

4 hours of sleep just 2 nights in a row, their levels of ghrelin increased by 28 percent, and their appetites by a whopping 23 percent, especially for salty snacks and sweets.

Tip: Sleep between 7 and 8 hours each night. To get that amount, keep your room dark, quiet, and cool, and develop a pre-sleep ritual, such as a 10-minute meditation, to banish the day's stresses.

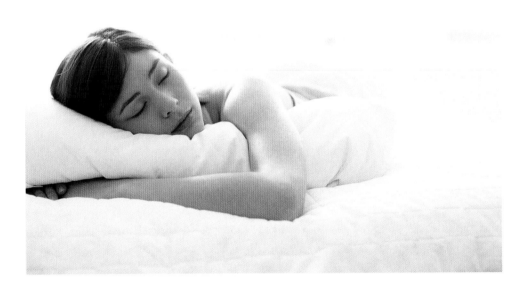

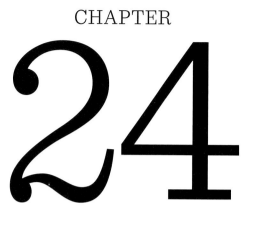

Boost Your
BRAINPOWER

Think sharper and look slimmer with our 7-day ultimate body-and-mind routine.

The road to a fit mind isn't paved in crossword puzzles alone. In fact, walking that road can also give your gray matter a boost, according to top researchers.

"Exercise is as close to a magic bullet as brain fitness gets," says John J. Medina, PhD, director of the Brain Center for Applied Learning Research at Seattle Pacific University. Physical activity bathes neural tissue in oxygen-rich blood, increasing the production of chemicals that improve memory, attention, and problem solving.

When sedentary adults in one study jogged for half an hour two or three times a week for 12 weeks, their memory and ability to juggle tasks improved by 30 percent. Just as important: Inactivity stops this process. When the participants returned to their couch potato ways, they lost 10 percent of the gain after 6 weeks.

To create the ultimate brainpower workout, we developed this 7-day plan based on cutting-edge research that will wake you up above the neck while still delivering the calorie-torching, body-toning benefits of ordinary workouts. The twist: Simple tweaks such as choosing scenic walking routes, closing your eyes while strength training, and even playing catch activate areas of your brain that regular exercise doesn't challenge. Follow along for a week's worth of workouts, then continue to use the strategies below as often as possible, whether you repeat the 7-day plan or incorporate the techniques into your own routine.

FOUR HABITS THAT BRIGHTEN YOUR BRAIN

What do smart people do to feel sharp for life? According to new research in *Neurology,* older adults who maintain their mental sharpness are more likely to have certain healthy traits than those who show decline. They exercise regularly, work or volunteer, have a high school degree and at least a ninth-grade literacy level, and don't smoke.

One theory: Exercising and not smoking allow more oxygen flow to the brain, while socializing and having an education strengthen connections between neurons, explains study author Alexandra Fiocco, PhD.

Day 1: Take a Nature Walk

Why it's a brain booster: University of Michigan researchers found that memory and attention improved by 20 percent when people walked in a park versus an urban environment. Natural settings have a restful effect, allowing the brain to process information better, explains study coauthor Marc Berman, a PhD candidate and psychology researcher. Busy surroundings—noisy traffic, colorful billboards, and throngs of people—clamor for

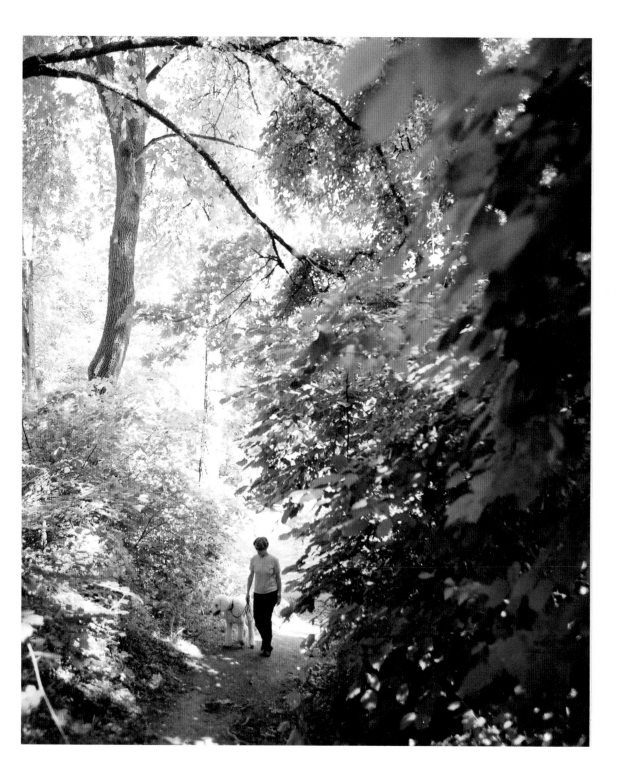

attention and distract you. An iPod can do the same, so leave it at home to emerge calmer, more focused—and better able to tackle your to-do list.

Day 2: Connect with Your Senses

Why it's a brain booster: Studies have long shown that tai chi improves balance. Now research demonstrates that it may also protect the area of the brain responsible for the sense of touch, which tends to fade rapidly after age 40.

In a recent Harvard study, 50- to 60-year-olds who did tai chi had more acute sensation in their fingertips, equivalent to that of people nearly half their age. Improved ability to feel can help you thread a needle, savor hugs from loved ones, or react quickly to a hot stove. As you age, it also helps prevent falls.

Tai chi's controlled movements strengthen nerve pathways to the fingers and toes, which become less responsive without practice, according to study author Catherine Kerr, PhD. Try it at www.prevention.com/taichi.

Day 3: Add in Speed

Why it's a brain booster: A 2007 study found that exercisers who did two 3-minute sprints memorized new words 20 percent faster afterward than those who skipped the workout. Cardio exercise increases blood flow, triggering growth in the area of the hippocampus responsible for memory and verbal learning, research shows. The proliferation of new brain cells might actually be linked to a bigger brain.

In a University of Pittsburgh study, the most aerobically fit had an average 7 percent larger hippocampus size than their sofa-sitting peers did. (A small hippocampus may be to blame for forgotten appointments or names.)

Day 4: Challenge Your Balance

Why it's a brain booster: Emerging research reveals a link between toning your muscles and toning your brain. In a Canadian study, older adults who lifted weights and also did walking and balance exercises improved their decision-making abilities by nearly 13 percent in 6 months. Adding a balance and coordination challenge to standard strength moves—such as simultaneously raising your right arm and left leg—might magnify the benefit.

"Complex movements force your mind to work harder by engaging multiple parts of the brain," says John Martin, PhD, a neuroscientist at Columbia University. Start with the following four mind-sharpening moves from Michael Gonzalez-Wallace, creator of the Brain Muscle Workout, which will also sculpt your arms, legs, back,

The percentage that risk of cognitive decline is reduced in people doing the most engaging leisure activities, according to researchers at the Albert Einstein School of Medicine:

54

and belly. Do 3 sets of 10 reps. Already lift weights? Add these moves to your regular workout to amp up brainpower and firm up faster.

Balancing arm raise: Stand, holding the dumbbells at your sides, palms back. Lift your right knee to hip height as you raise your left arm up in front, elbow straight, until it's overhead. Lower your arm and switch sides.

Ballerina curl: Stand with your feet wide, toes out, holding the dumbbells at your sides, palms forward. Bend your knees, lowering your hips. As you stand, curl the dumbbells toward your shoulders and lift your heels. Lower the dumbbells, then your heels, and repeat.

Coordination crunch: Lie on your back with a dumbbell in each hand near your chest, with your elbows bent out to the sides, legs extended over your hips, and abs tight. Simultaneously open your legs into a V as you lift your head and shoulders off the floor and press the weights straight up over your chest. Lower to the start position, bringing your legs together, and repeat.

Step and pull: Stand with your left foot about 3 feet in front of the right, the dumbbells at your sides, palms back. Bend your knees to lower into a lunge, your front knee over your ankle. Stand, bending your elbows out to the sides to pull the weights up to chest level, and bring your right knee forward to hip height. Balance, then step back into another lunge, lowering your arms.

Day 5: Toss a Ball while Walking

Why it's a brain booster: German researchers found that adolescents who bounced, threw, or passed balls with alternating hands for just 10 minutes increased their attention and concentration in a subsequent lesson and test. You don't have to be a kid to benefit, say study authors, who

The percentage of women who crave chocolate when they "need a pick-me-up," according to a 2007 ConAgra Foods Survey:

58

2-Minute Memory Trick

Constantly forget where you parked? Breathing through your left nostril may help, say Indian researchers. Adults ages 20 to 45 who practiced this yoga technique had a 16 percent boost in spatial memory, which is key for navigating complex parking lots or garages. Experts believe there's a link between the nostril you breathe through and parts of the brain that control memory.

Try this: Gently press your right thumb against your right nostril. Inhale and exhale through your left nostril 27 times. Repeat up to four times a day.

speculate that handling a ball primes the part of the brain that controls focus.

Day 6: Repeat Day 3— With a Friend

Why it's a brain booster: A substantial body of research suggests that beefing up your social calendar decreases your chances of memory loss. A study in the *American Journal of Public Health* reported that women with large social networks slashed their risk of dementia by as much as 26 percent. Plus, psychology research concludes that encouraging others to exercise will ensure that you follow through, too.

Day 7: Repeat Day 4— With Your Eyes Closed

Why it's a brain booster: "When you take away visual cues, you push your brain to use circuits that aren't normally engaged," says Dr. Martin. Your brain relies on a com-

THE SWEETEST WAY TO STAY FOCUSED

Dig into dark chocolate to beat brain fog! Cocoa flavanols—phytonutrients abundant in dark chocolate—might keep the brain alert by increasing blood flow, according to research presented at the British Psychological Society's annual conference. When adults consumed a drink containing cocoa flavanols, they reported less mental fatigue.

For a brain boost, sip a cup of dark chocolate hot cocoa—we like Green & Black's Organic Hot Chocolate Drink. Or nibble on a few small squares of dark chocolate containing at least 70 percent cacao.

bination of sensory information from your limbs, joints, and eyes to coordinate movements. By closing your eyes, you force your brain to adapt. This improves plasticity, which is your mind's ability to change and refine when faced with new experiences, a process that tends to wane with age.

BE HAPPY

Live in the "sunshine state." Happiness, even in trying times, is very much under your control. **Here are eye-opening ways to ensure that it never eludes your grasp.**

The year 2010 was one that few of us will soon forget. But the tough times we've been through illuminate the human ability to weather challenges that at first might seem overwhelming. As so many millions have painfully learned, we can't fully control our circumstances. Surprisingly often, though, we can control their effects on our well-being.

Experts attribute about 50 percent of our individual happiness to genetic endowments and another 10 percent to circumstances—where we live, how much money we make, how healthy we are. That leaves 40 percent of our happiness within our control. Fortunately, science has much to say about how we can make the most of that 40 percent. Even small improvements in mood can have cascading effects. The trick is to pay attention to which strategies work best for you. Try these for starters.

Know What to Want

Most of us can't predict what will make us happy in the future, and that inability often leads us down the wrong path.

"The average American moves more than 11 times, changes jobs more than 10 times, and marries more than once, suggesting that most of us are making more than a few poor choices," says Harvard University psychologist Daniel Gilbert, PhD, author of *Stumbling on Happiness.*

One reason we so often guess wrong, he argues, is that we often imagine the future incorrectly. We forget how easily we adapt

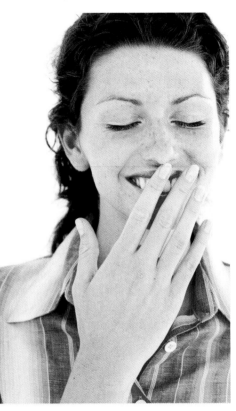

even to painful circumstances. So when we picture what it would be like to be single again or to live in Seattle or to leave one job for another, we don't factor in everything else—the new friends, the newly discovered interest in Cascade Mountains wildflowers—that might also affect our emotional well-being. Unfortunately, Dr. Gilbert notes, we can't simply train ourselves to peer into the future with greater clarity. Instead we should put more trust in other people's experiences.

"Start with the assumption that your reactions are a lot like other people's," he says. If you want to know whether to take a job at a new company, pay attention to the people around you when you're there for an interview. Do they seem engaged and interested? That should count for a lot.

Savor Mystery

In a culture obsessed with the power of information, the fact that most of us are a little unnerved by uncertainty is hardly surprising. Yet research suggests that a dash of mystery can make positive experiences last longer.

In one study, University of Virginia psychologist Timothy D. Wilson, PhD, and his colleagues found that students who were given a $1 coin with little explanation reported feeling happier a few minutes later than those who were given either the same amount of money by a known source or no money at all. Dr. Wilson argues that those who didn't fully comprehend the reason for the gift spent more time mulling it over, extending their pleasure.

"Once we've done the cognitive work to understand something, we kind of wrap it up in a little package and store it away and move on to other things," he explains. It's not easy to stage surprises for yourself, but Dr. Wilson suggests a few tricks. Next time you're nearing the end of an engrossing book, save the final pages for a few days later. Or shop from catalogs so you won't know exactly when your purchases will arrive. If you're lucky, when they do you may have forgotten what you ordered.

Hope for Small Changes, Not Big Ones

Research shows that even major life events, such as winning the lottery, hardly nudge people's overall sense of satisfaction. But that doesn't mean you shouldn't try to improve your well-being. Recent research finds that the little things we do regularly, such as exercising or attending religious services, can have a major impact on our happiness.

In one study, Yale University psychologist Daniel Mochon, PhD, and his colleagues at Harvard and Duke universities discovered that people leaving religious services felt slightly happier than those going in, and the more regularly people attended religious services, the happier they felt overall. The same is true for exercise. People feel happier after going to the gym or to a yoga class, and they also get a bigger boost the more often they go.

In Kindness, Seek Variety

Being kind and helpful makes most everyone feel good. But just as the novelty of a new car or electronic gadget inevitably wears off, so does the warm glow that comes from doing the same good deed over and over.

People who performed various small acts of kindness every week for 10 weeks—shoveling a friend's sidewalk, giving pets a special treat, sending a birthday card—grew happier with each passing week, and the benefit lasted for at least another month, found a study by psychology professor Sonja Lyubomirsky, PhD, and her colleagues at the University of California, Riverside. In contrast, people who did the same kind act repeatedly became less happy after a few weeks, then reverted to their prior level of contentment.

Try this: Do several good deeds in 1 day; researchers say your happiness boost will be greater than if you spread them out evenly over time.

Shift Your Focus

From work to relationships to health, we have choices about where to concentrate our attention. When a snowstorm keeps you from getting to the office, do you choose to focus on how behind you'll be by tomorrow, or do you focus on the 8-hour gift of time you've just been given? When you paint your daughter's bedroom, do you fret about how much you hate the drudgery, or

think ahead to how pleased she'll be when she comes home for Christmas break?

The answer to such questions has a big influence on your well-being, writes Winifred Gallagher, author of *Rapt: Attention and the Focused Life*. Studies show that focusing on positive emotions—curiosity instead of fear, compassion instead of anger—leads to broader, more flexible thinking, more playfulness and exploration, and richer social connections. Positive emotions also temper negative feelings' corrosive physiological effects—especially their impact on the cardiovascular system.

It's not surprising, then, that people who habitually adopt an optimistic focus have fewer health problems and live longer than their more pessimistic counterparts.

Let Your Mind Wander

The flip side of focus is daydreaming. Although we spend up to one-third of our waking lives in this luscious state of "undirected thought," we often dismiss daydreaming as a sign of procrastination and laziness. But recent brain-imaging research shows that when you're daydreaming, your brain is actually working pretty hard.

In one recent study, University of British Columbia psychologist Kalina Christoff, PhD, and her colleagues found that people who allowed their minds to wander while doing simple tasks tapped into not only their "executive" brain network

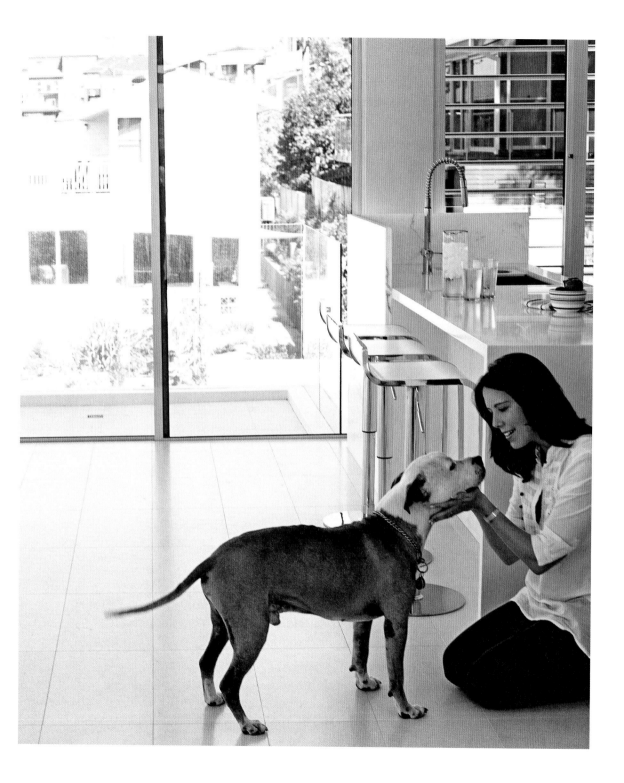

(source of logical thinking and problem solving) but also their "default network," which is the wellspring for creative thought and relaxed, introspective thinking. To rev brainpower, Dr. Christoff suggests alternating deliberate, focused thinking with more spontaneous mind wandering. Another strategy is to occasionally set aside time for uninterrupted daydreaming, like a stolen hour for a walk in the park.

Know When to Fold 'Em

Most of us are not very good at knowing when to walk away from circumstances that are just plain bad—a human foible that economists and psychologists call the fallacy of sunk costs. We keep holding when we should be folding—sticking with bad jobs because of the months and years we've already sunk into them, unhappy relationships that we can't imagine extracting ourselves from, or sluggish supermarket lines we've stood in too long to abandon.

Because we're so averse to wasting money, time, effort, or emotional investment, we fail to see that staying the course won't recoup what we've already lost, observes Hal Arkes, PhD, a psychology professor at the Ohio State University in Columbus. But this is a failure we can overcome by deliberately thinking through our choices as though we weren't already invested in one course of action. The next time you're faced with a problem that has gone from good to bad to worse, think to yourself, *If I were coming into this situation right now, what would I do?*

Give Money Away

Once a person's basic needs are met, having more money does little to boost happiness, studies show. What matters more is how much you give away.

In a survey of 632 Americans, University of British Columbia psychologist Elizabeth Dunn, PhD, and her colleagues found that the money people spent on themselves was unrelated to general happiness, but the more money people gave away as gifts and donations, the happier they were.

In another study, the researchers gave people $5 or $20 with instructions to spend the money on themselves, spend it on someone else, or donate it. Those who gave the money away or spent it on others—no matter the amount—were happier than those who used it for themselves.

Talk to Your Spouse Like a Stranger

No one wants to make a bad first impression, so we tend to put our best face forward, especially with people we don't know. And that turns out to be a good strategy for enhancing our own happiness.

In one study, Dr. Dunn and her colleagues learned that people conversing with strangers tried harder to make good impressions than did people conversing with their romantic partners, and the more they did so, the happier they felt after the interaction was over.

Another experiment showed that people instructed to talk with their romantic partners as though they were trying to make a good impression (as they would with a stranger) felt happier after the experiment ended than those who were told to interact normally.

Settle for Good Enough

We tend to equate choice with freedom—and what could be wrong with that? Plenty, according to Swarthmore College psychologist Barry Schwartz, PhD, author of *The Paradox of Choice.*

Faced with a vast array of options—whether among consumer products like blue jeans and toothpastes or more consequential services like prescription drug plans and retirement plans—many of us end up bewildered. We can't stop worrying that what we don't choose might make us happier. One simple solution, Dr. Schwartz argues, is to opt out of the multiple-choice game by narrowing your pick to several "good enough" options—then choose randomly.

Make Something

Few activities are as reliably pleasurable as making things with our own hands. In one study, Harvard University psychologist Michael I. Norton, PhD, and his colleagues asked participants to make origami, then to bid on their artwork along with others. People were willing to pay more for their own amateurish work than for others' attempts—and in many cases, they rated their creations as more valuable than origami made by professionals.

One catch: To get the boost in satisfaction that comes from making something—whether an origami crane or a new coffee table—you need to actually finish the job. Alas, a lovely knitted sweater with one sleeve won't give you the same emotional boost.

AVOID

Here's how to ward off diabetes complications

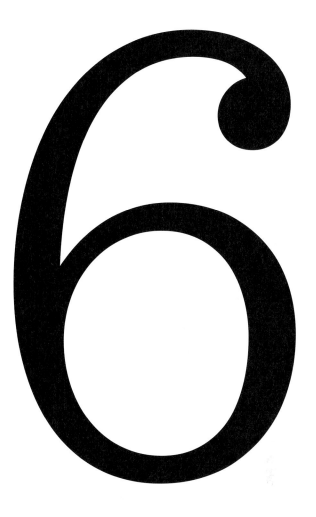

PART

COMPLICATIONS

and keep them from complicating you.

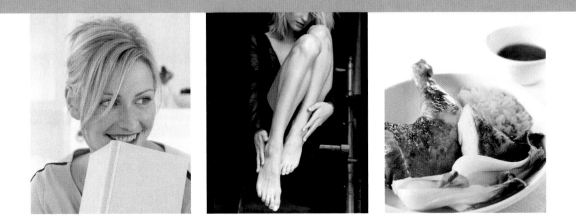

COMPLICATIONS
Medical Breakthroughs

Life with diabetes is anything but simple. In addition to controlling your blood sugar to keep your diabetes in check, you have to keep its many complications at bay. People with diabetes are at increased risk of high blood pressure, heart disease, cancer, erectile dysfunction, and even Alzheimer's disease.

MAXIMIZE YOUR MEMORY: ALLITERATE!

To better remember a to-do list item, try creating an alliteration, which is a phrase that contains repeated consonant sounds, such as "Purchase pretty produce." Researchers had subjects read poetry and prose both silently and aloud. Later, participants recalled passages containing alliterative phrases much better than they did others.

Researcher Brooke Lea, PhD, of Macalester College in St. Paul, Minnesota, suggests keeping the phrases simple. Ones like "exercise at eight" or "dial the doctor" may even augment your healthy lifestyle.

FIGHT DEMENTIA

Here are three key ways.

Lower your cholesterol: People at high risk of dementia who took a statin for 5 years were half as likely to develop the condition as those who weren't on the drug, a University of Michigan study shows.

Choose the right blood pressure med: Taking angiotensin II receptor blockers cut the risk of dementia by up to 40 percent, compared with ACE inhibitors or other hypertension drugs, Boston University scientists found.

Try hypnosis: Among dementia patients, it improved concentration, relaxation, memory, and social skills better than standard treatment, say researchers at the United Kingdom's University of Liverpool.

PROTECT YOUR BRAIN

Eat more chicken. It might help, thanks to a little-publicized nutrient that seems to prevent memory loss associated with Alzheimer's disease, according to a new study. When researchers gave mice with dementia nicotinamide (a form of B_3, or niacin), they performed memory tasks as if they'd never had the disease. The vitamin also boosted memory in normal mice.

Scientists believe B_3 lowers levels of a protein that contributes to tangles that can clog brain cells and lead to Alzheimer's. Be sure to get around 14 milligrams of B_3 a day, which is the amount in a serving of chicken and $1/2$ cup of brown rice.

WORRY ABOUT YOURSELF

People take heart attack symptoms more seriously in others than in themselves, according to a British Heart Foundation survey. Even though 47 percent of people would tell a parent having unusual chest pain to call for an ambulance, 65 percent would not call if they experienced the same symptoms.

TREAT YOUR FEET

Relief is just a step away for the 75 percent of Americans who are prone to foot pain: CrocsRx, a line of ergonomic clogs and socks, promises to ease a number of foot ailments, including those caused by arthritis, heel spurs, plantar fasciitis, and poor circulation. The Custom Cloud model is ideal for people with diabetes,

The percentage of older adults who worry about their memory abilities, according to a 2007 Alzheimer's Association of America survey:

73

offering extra protection and custom moldable inserts. All of the models have been accepted by the American Podiatric Medical Association.

▓ FIX YOUR FOOT PAIN

Surgery is a last resort for treating bunions, painful bumps on the sides of big toes (blame age, heredity, or high heels), but the Bunion Aid splint may delay the need for an operation indefinitely. You can wear the flexible splint 24-7 and inside shoes (unlike standard rigid splints, which are worn only at night).

In a German study of bunion patients whose big toes were off line by an average of 29 degrees, a night splint reduced the misalignment to 18 degrees, but the Bunion Aid splint lowered it to nearly 11 degrees (www.alphaorthotics.com).

▓ DON'T WAIT IN "VEIN"

Roughly 20 percent of Americans have varicose veins in their legs, often accompanied by pain. Yet 87 percent of people with this condition have never had it examined by a doctor. This is especially risky business for people with diabetes.

Unfortunately, people don't consider varicose veins to be a serious issue, according to a Vein Clinics of America survey. Yet varicose veins are often more than just a cosmetic nuisance. Severe ones might put you at risk for leg ulcers, bleeding, and clots, so always get them checked out.

26

Improve Your Habits,
IMPROVE YOUR HEALTH

The rewards of starting a good habit (or mending a bad one) **come quicker than you think.**

Remember those healthy resolutions you made earlier this year? If you need a little extra motivation to stick to them, try this: According to recent research, adults who quit smoking, ate more fruits and veggies, exercised a few hours a week, and watched their weight significantly slashed their risk of cardiovascular disease (and of any disease-related death) in just 4 years. And cardiovascular disease is one of many complications of diabetes.

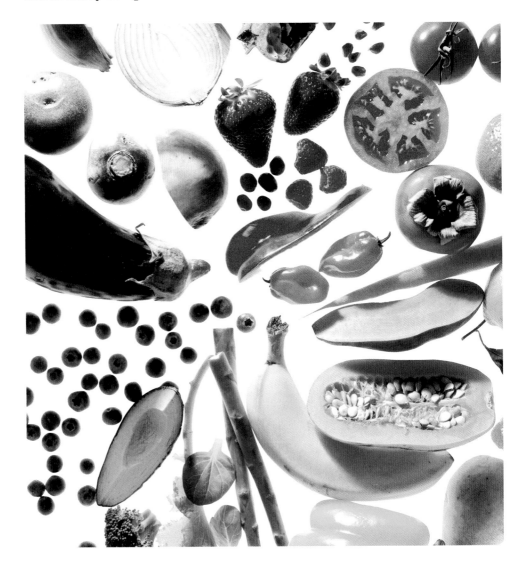

It's never too late to clean up your act. Adopt the same behaviors, and your health will improve as dramatically; keep at it, and the benefits multiply. Here, four habits to start (or break) and how quickly you'll see the results of your efforts.

Quit Smoking

Improves health in 1 day.

Quitting smoking won't affect your diabetes directly, but it will help your heart and lungs—and it lowers the risk of damage to your blood vessels, eyes, nerves, and other organs. Plus, quitting smoking can leave you with fewer wrinkles; better-smelling hair, breath, and clothes; and less exposure for your family to secondhand smoke.

Within 20 minutes after you finish your last cigarette, your heart rate and blood pressure (revved by the nicotine in tobacco) start to drop. Within 12 hours, toxic carbon monoxide, or CO, in your blood from the cigarette smoke decreases and oxygen levels increase, improving cell health and circulation. This is key because just a 1 percent rise in carbon monoxide levels in your blood ups your risk of tobacco-related death by 22 percent.

If you stay smoke free for around 2 months, research shows, you can lower CO levels by up to 17 percent.

Lung function also improves in about 2 weeks. The tiny brushlike structures in your lungs called cilia (which sweep away pollen and dust and keep your lungs clear) begin to repair themselves, reducing your risk of breathing problems and cell damage, explains Bill Blatt, MPH, director of tobacco programs for the American Lung Association.

Within 5 to 10 years, the risk of dying from respiratory disease is cut by 18 percent; from lung cancer, by 21 percent. Even if your lungs have been damaged, quitting helps: Among nearly 6,000 middle-aged smokers with mild lung disease, quitters had a 46 percent lower death rate over 14.5 years than those who kept lighting up, according to a 2005 study.

GET STARTED

It takes most people seven to nine tries to succeed, so hang in there.

"You need to find the right combination of methods," says Blatt, which might include relaxation techniques, setting up a support system, and medication. Talk with your primary care physician, or contact your local American Lung Association branch.

Eat More Fruits and Veggies

Improves health in 14 days.

Eating fruits and vegetables is important for everyone, but possibly even more so for people with diabetes. One of the many benefits is that produce gives you plenty of fiber, which slows the rate at which sugar enters your bloodstream and might reduce spikes in blood sugar levels.

Produce is also loaded with nutrients that might lower blood pressure, including potassium, magnesium, calcium, and antioxidants. That's why fruits and vegetables are the cornerstone of the DASH (Dietary Approaches to Stop Hypertension) diet. Researchers found that upping produce intake and switching to low-fat dairy products lowered systolic blood pressure (the upper number in blood pressure readings) by nearly six points and diastolic (the lower number) by three points in 2 weeks—almost as much as medication can achieve. Reducing sodium intake as well—to just 1,500 milligrams per day, or about $2/3$ teaspoon—can shave another five and three points, respectively.

Hypertension forces the heart to work harder to circulate blood, explains Daniel W. Jones, MD, a hypertension specialist and chancellor of the University of Mississippi. Over time, that causes damage to blood vessels and arteries, which might lead to kidney or heart disease.

In fact, a published meta-analysis found that individuals who ate more than five servings of fruits and vegetables per day had roughly a 20 percent lower risk of coronary heart disease, compared with people who ate fewer than three servings per day. According to the Nurses' Health Study, following a diet that lowers blood pressure, maintaining a healthy weight, and exercising regularly might help prevent 53 percent of new cases of hypertension in women at risk.

GET STARTED

To up your intake of fresh produce to five or more servings per day, try these simple strategies: Keep your favorite fruits visible, such as in a bowl on the kitchen counter. If you see them regularly, you'll be more likely to eat them. One serving of fruit equates to one medium apple or banana or $1/2$ cup of canned fruit.

Also, make sure half of your plate is filled with a vegetable at every meal. One serving equals 1 cup of raw leafy vegetables or $1/2$ cup of another vegetable, such as baby carrots or corn.

For more information on the DASH diet—which also recommends six servings of whole grains; three to six of lean meat, poultry, and fish; and two of fats and oils, for 1,600 calories a day—see www.prevention.com/links.

Exercise 60 Minutes Every Week

Improves health in 90 days.

Exercise is critical for people with diabetes. It can help you improve your blood sugar control and also reduce your risk of complications, such as heart disease.

Older women who walked at a moderate pace for 20 minutes three times a week for 3 months improved their aerobic fitness by 12 percent, according to research conducted by *Prevention* advisor Wayne L. Westcott, PhD, fitness research director at Quincy College in Massachusetts. Participants also lowered their resting

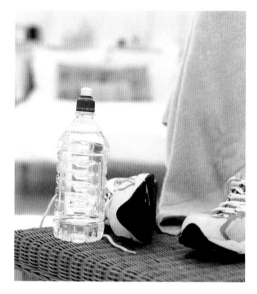

heart rate from 75 beats per minute (bpm) to 68. Most people have resting heart rates between 60 and 80 bpm. The closer your rate is to 60, the healthier your heart.

You can achieve additional health benefits with a more taxing regimen: Australian scientists found that adults who did at least three 60-minute sessions of intensive activities (such as resistance training or Spinning) every week for about a month saw a 16 percent improvement in aerobic fitness, which signifies better heart health and muscle endurance. They also lowered their cholesterol and blood glucose levels as well as weight, body mass index, and waist circumference and reported feeling more energetic, points out Lynda Norton, PhD, lead author and research associate at Flinders University of South Australia.

In addition, researchers at Washington University in St. Louis School of Medi-cine found that 1 hour of vigorous walking or cycling 5 days a week can reverse age-related deterioration of your heart's function after 7 months.

GET STARTED

"The best exercise is the one you'll do," says Steven N. Blair, PED, a professor of exercise science at the University of South Carolina in Columbia.

Choose any activity you enjoy—be it walking, cycling, or dancing—and aim for a minimum of 20 to 25 minutes a day. Break it down, if you have to, into two 10-minute sessions. Slowly increase the frequency, duration, and intensity. If you miss a day, pick up again the next day, but still try to meet the weekly total. And if you want to track the benefits of your program to your resting heart rate, lay a finger on your wrist to find your pulse, count the number of beats in 15 seconds, and then multiply it by 4 to get your resting rate per minute.

Cut Saturated Fat

Improves health in 90 to 180 days.

Reducing saturated fat helps lower cholesterol, which not only lowers your risk of heart disease and stroke but also keeps your brain healthy. A recent 40-year study of nearly 10,000 people found that having high cholesterol increases the risk of Alzheimer's disease by 57 percent. Even borderline-high levels raise vascular dementia risk by 50 percent.

Because both heart disease and Alzheimer's disease go hand in hand with diabetes, this is especially important for people with diabetes.

"Saturated fat helps produce unhealthy LDL cholesterol," says Vincent J. Bufalino, MD, a Chicago-based cardiologist and spokesperson for the American Heart Association. Too much LDL in your system, and it begins to build up in the arteries that transport blood to your heart and brain. Over time, LDL cholesterol turns into plaque that hardens, narrowing arteries and making them less pliable.

GET STARTED

The more saturated fat you cut from your diet—regardless of your age—the more your LDL drops, according to a study published in an American Heart Association journal. Limit saturated fat to 7 percent of your daily calories (that's about 112 calories for a 1,600-calorie day, or roughly 12 grams of saturated fat) and you can lower your LDL by about 10 percent.

Here are some guidelines to help you cut saturated fat and lower cholesterol: Eat red meat no more than twice a week, switch to fat-free milk, and increase your fiber intake to 20 to 25 grams daily, which can lower LDL by up to another 10 percent, advises Dr. Bufalino. If you make these tweaks to your diet, your cholesterol should begin to improve in 3 to 6 months.

27

Prevent the Problem

MEN DREAD

Erectile dysfunction is a leading indicator of heart trouble, and a complication of diabetes. **Keep your romance healthy with our tips.**

Turn on the television, and you'll likely see an ad hyping erection-boosting drugs. But erectile dysfunction, or ED, is a health issue that's rarely mentioned in any other context. It should be—and not for the obvious reasons. Although an injury or a psychological trigger such as depression can cause ED, many studies show that repeated difficulty having or sustaining an erection is a serious indicator of heart trouble, especially with age.

The percentage of people who say they brush and floss less when they're stressed, according to the *Journal of Periodontology:*

56

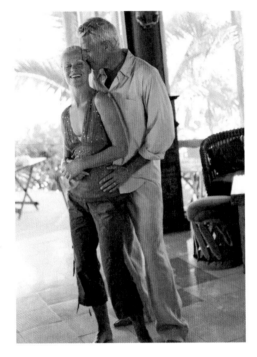

"When a man walks into a doctor's office complaining of erection problems, chances are his heart is in trouble as well," says Irwin Goldstein, MD, director of sexual medicine at Alvarado Hospital in San Diego.

Urologist Ian M. Thompson, MD, of the University of Texas Health Science Center at San Antonio, revealed the extent of the problem when he reported in the *Journal of the American Medical Association* (*JAMA*) that men ages 55 and older with ED have a 55 percent greater risk of developing cardiovascular disease, resulting in a heart attack or stroke, than men without this problem.

The ED-diabetes connection is also clear. One study found that 50 percent of males with type 2 diabetes have ED. Other studies have found that men with diabetes have lower testosterone levels, which affects libido.

The older a man gets, the more likely he'll experience ED. Prevalence soars from 9 percent in 40-something men to 15 percent for those in their fifties, and 29 percent for those between 60 and 69, according to a study in the *Journal of Sexual Medicine.* If you or your partner is experiencing ED, it's important to review heart health with a primary care physician and perhaps visit a cardiologist as well.

Heart health and ED are linked because both depend on tiny arteries. Vessels in the penis, which deliver the blood that causes this organ to expand, are just as susceptible to narrowing and clogging as those in a man's heart, explains Dr. Goldstein. Because penile arteries are smaller than those in the heart, they're often the first to show the effects of bad habits, such as smoking and eating fatty foods.

If a man's ED means he has heart issues, his cardiologist may okay Viagra or other ED drugs if the cardiac problems are not extensive, states Dr. Thompson. Who can't use them: men with serious heart disease and those who take nitrate medicines. (Men with diabetes can use ED drugs but may find they don't work well.)

Medication isn't the only choice, though. Experts say that lifestyle changes can improve ED and even reverse it in some cases, and they'll certainly do any man's heart good. Here are five options.

Lose weight: Simply shedding pounds allowed one-third of obese midlife men with ED to regain, within 2 years, their ability to have an erection, reported Italian scientists in *JAMA*. The extra weight restricts blood flow and increases inflammation in blood vessels, upping the risk of both ED and heart disease. The researchers say that the men in the study reversed these changes by cutting calories to about 1,700 per day during the first year of the study and to 1,900 after that. They also exercised—walking, swimming, or playing aerobic sports such as soccer—for about 3 hours per week.

Start moving: No matter what a man's weight is, exercise can help solve ED issues, according to Elizabeth Selvin, PhD, MPH, an assistant professor of epidemiology and medicine at the Johns Hopkins Bloomberg School of Public Health in Baltimore. The more energetic the activity, the better. After analyzing a nationwide health-and-nutrition survey, she reported that men who work out vigorously have an ED risk of just 10 percent. In contrast, moderate exercisers more than double their risk (22 percent). Sedentary men hit 26 percent. But beware: If the exercise a man chooses is bicycling, he should use a wide, noseless seat, not a long, narrow one, researchers say. Narrow seats press on the groin's nerves and blood vessels, affecting blood supply to the penis.

Stop smoking: According to Dr. Thompson, smokers have a 60 percent higher risk of ED. "Smoking affects the ability of blood vessels to expand and produce an erection," he explains. Nearly 23 percent of ED in Chinese men ages 35 to 74 was linked to

BRUSH UP YOUR SEX LIFE

Men who are lax about tooth care may also have trouble becoming sexually aroused. Israeli researchers found that more than 15 percent of men with moderate to severe erectile dysfunction had chronic gum disease, compared with only 2 percent of men without ED. Oral bacteria travel through the bloodstream, attaching to plaque and narrowing vessels in the penis, which supply blood for erections. Brush twice and floss once a day for a healthy mouth—and a satisfying sex life.

Prevent the Problem

Simply put: Have more sex. Think of the penis as a muscle that needs regular workouts to stay in shape, advise Finnish researchers. They announced in 2008 that men ages 55 to 75 who had intercourse less than once a week, on average, were twice as likely to develop ED as men who had intercourse weekly. One possible reason: Just as the increased blood flow produced by aerobic exercise keeps heart arteries pliable and healthy, regular intercourse keeps the blood vessels in the penis in good working order.

cigarette smoking, report experts at Tulane University. And the more a man lit up, the more problems he experienced: Those who smoked up to 10 cigarettes per day had a 27 percent greater chance of developing ED, while those who smoked more than 20 cigarettes daily were 65 percent more likely to have the condition.

Cut back on alcohol: Even a drink or two can affect some men's ability to have and sustain an erection. An analysis published in the *International Journal of Impotence Research* in 2007 found that downing eight or more drinks per week seems to raise the risk of ED, though the reason is unclear.

Start talking: For some men with ED, it's not all physiology. Psychological issues may also be to blame, and talking can help. According to a Cochrane Collaboration Systematic Review, 95 percent of the men in a psychotherapy group who discussed their ED with fellow sufferers said good-bye to persistent problems with erectile dysfunction, while others without treatment had no improvement. A man can find a group with the assistance of his physician or a therapist.

28

Beat High Blood
PRESSURE

Here's how to beat hypertension, aka high blood pressure, which often goes hand in hand with diabetes.

I n an eerie parallel, just as people often feel no symptoms when their blood sugar levels rise, many people also feel no different when their blood pressure rises. To make matters worse, high blood pressure often accompanies diabetes.

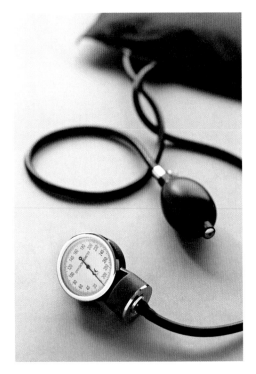

How high is too high? Most people should aim to keep their blood pressure below 130/88 mm Hg.

Having high blood pressure increases your risk of heart attack and stroke. One of the most preventable diseases, hypertension plays a contributing role in more than 15 percent of deaths in the United States, according to a new Harvard study. Fortunately, most people can reduce it without medication. First get to a healthy weight. Then add these strategies.

Check It Often

A blood pressure monitor is "a must-have for everyone over 40," says John Elefteriades, MD, chief of cardiothoracic surgery at Yale University School of Medicine. High blood pressure has no symptoms, and if you don't know you have it, you can't bring it down—an achievement that cuts your risk of stroke in half and reduces your heart attack risk by 25 percent.

If your blood pressure hasn't been a problem in the past, check it once a month; if you have high blood pressure, check it weekly. Report to your doctor values that are consistently greater than 140/90, advises Dr. Elefteriades.

Most doctors now support the idea of self-checking your blood pressure, but the accuracy of home monitors can vary widely, according to recent tests on 16 models by researchers at *Consumer Reports*. Fortunately, reliability is not necessarily dependent on price, they found— one of the best performers was less than half the cost of other top-notch models. The following monitors received high marks for accuracy and overall value.

Omron Women's Advanced Elite 7300W: Top-rated overall, this monitor includes an irregular-heartbeat detector.

Omron Automatic with IntelliSense HEM-711AC: Very accurate and slightly cheaper, it has fewer extra features.

Tip: Measure your upper-arm circumference before buying so you know your cuff size. Using the correct cuff ensures more accurate readings.

Consider Your History

This one is for women only: Think back to your pregnancy. If you had high blood pressure or preeclampsia, you should be extra vigilant about having your blood pressure checked and controlled. Women who had hypertension while pregnant had symptoms of heart disease about 3 years sooner than women with normal blood pressure.

Women who had gestational diabetes (GD) also have up to a 50 percent chance of developing type 2 diabetes within 10 years. If you had GD, tell your doc. You should get tested annually.

Schedule a Reminder

Whether you need to check your blood pressure weekly or daily, it might help you to schedule reminders. A study found that patients were 16 percent more likely to schedule health screenings when they received a mailed reminder.

Send yourself an "e-nudge" for important tests, like blood pressure checks, at www.myhealthtestreminder.org, which is a new service from the College of American Pathologists.

Beat BP with Tea

Lowering blood pressure is as easy as one, two, tea: Study participants who sipped 3 cups of a hibiscus tea daily lowered systolic blood pressure by seven points in 6 weeks, on average, say researchers from Tufts University—results on a par with many prescription medications. Those who received a placebo drink improved their reading by only one point.

The phytochemicals in hibiscus are probably responsible for the large reduction, the study authors explain. Many herbal teas contain hibiscus. Look for blends that have it near the top of the list of ingredients; this often indicates a higher concentration per serving.

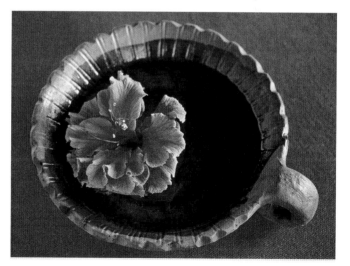

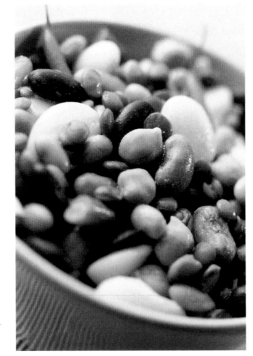

The percentage of first-time stroke patients whose blood pressure was above normal, according to the American Heart Association:

77

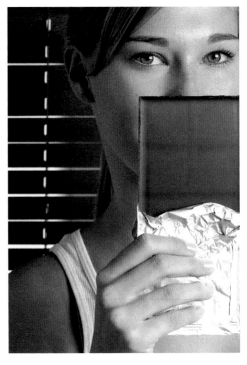

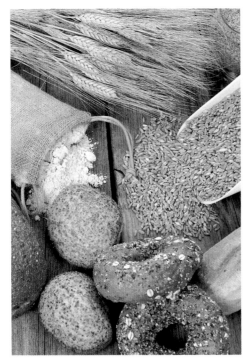

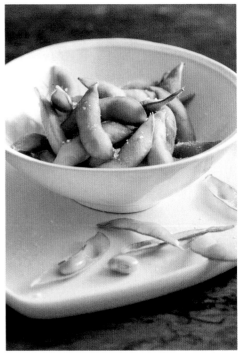

Go Pro(tein)

A diet rich in beans, whole grains, and soy products may help keep blood pressure in check. In a study of 4,680 adults, scientists found that a 5 percent higher intake of glutamic acid—the predominant amino acid in these nonanimal sources of protein—helped reduce blood pressure by up to 4.1 total points.

To increase your glutamic acid intake, eat like a vegetarian once a week: Choose a black bean burger over beef, or stir-fry tofu instead of pork.

Eat More Chocolate (Hurray!)

Dark varieties contain flavanols that make blood vessels more elastic. In one study, 18 percent of patients who ate it every day saw their blood pressure decrease.

Here's your Rx: Have 1/2 ounce daily of at least 70 percent cocoa.

Try These Power Pairs

If you have high blood pressure, pay attention to potassium. It helps the kidneys excrete surplus sodium from the body, thereby regulating blood pressure. Adults need about 4,700 milligrams per day, so load up on bananas and try these potassium-packed combos. (If you're taking blood pressure medication, consult with your doctor before increasing potassium.)

Power Pairs: Baked potato (1 medium) + kidney beans (1/2 cup)
Potassium (milligrams): 1,254
For a bigger boost: Mix in 1/2 cup cooked corn (111 milligrams).

Power Pairs: Fat-free milk (1 cup) + papaya (1 peeled, cubed)
Potassium (milligrams): 808
For a bigger boost: Sprinkle with 2 tablespoons ground flaxseed (114 milligrams).

Power Pairs: Quinoa (1 cup, cooked) + black beans (1/2 cup, cooked)
Potassium (milligrams): 623
For a bigger boost: Top with 1 large tomato, chopped (431 milligrams).

Power Pairs: Low-fat yogurt (1 cup) + walnuts (1/4 cup)
Potassium (milligrams): 544
For a bigger boost: Add 1 ounce raisins (212 milligrams).

Supplement

In a review of a dozen studies, researchers found that coenzyme Q10 reduced blood pressure by up to 17 mm Hg over 10 mm Hg. The antioxidant, required for energy production, dilates blood vessels.

Ask your doctor about taking a 60- to 100-milligram supplement up to three times a day.

Take a Power Walk

People with high blood pressure who walked at a brisk pace lowered pressure by almost 8 mm Hg over 6 mm Hg. Exercise helps the heart use oxygen more efficiently, so it doesn't work as hard to pump blood.

Get a vigorous cardio workout lasting at least 30 minutes on most days of the week. Try increasing speed or distance so you keep challenging your ticker.

Just Breathe

Alternate-nostril breathing—common in yoga—can reduce blood pressure by activating nasal receptors that calm your nervous system. In a recent study, people who did it twice a day for 3 months had readings up to 18 total points lower. Slow breathing and meditative practices such as qigong, yoga, and tai chi decrease stress hormones, which elevate renin, a kidney enzyme that raises blood pressure.

Here's how to do it: Close your right nostril with your thumb and inhale through your left nostril for 6 seconds. Release your thumb, close your left nostril with your index finger, and exhale for 6 seconds. Repeat for 3 minutes, working up to 15 minutes (the duration in the study) twice daily.

Or simply try 5 minutes of deep breathing in the morning and at night. Inhale deeply and expand your belly. Exhale and release all of your tension.

29

FIGHT CANCER

These medical professionals treat the disease—and they've all had it themselves. **Here's how cancer survivors say you can stay healthy.**

Surviving cancer was a life-changing experience for these top cancer experts, even though they'd spent their careers helping patients fight the illness—and thought they knew everything they needed to know to beat the disease.

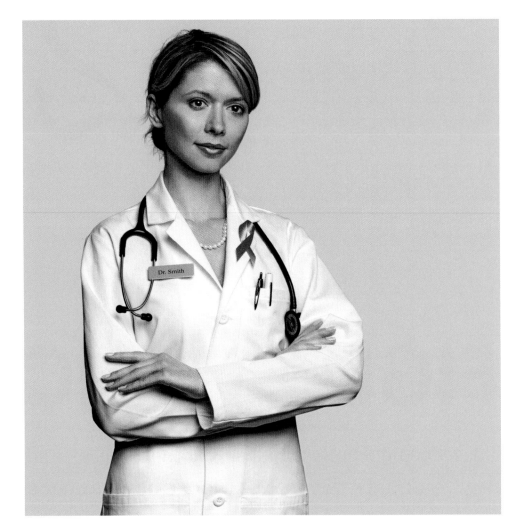

"When you're the patient, you learn a lot about what it really takes to keep yourself healthy," admits Carolyn D. Runowicz, MD, director of the Carole and Ray Neag Comprehensive Cancer Center at the University of Connecticut in Farmington. "Things like eating well and exercising regularly suddenly seem like a matter of life and death."

Here, she and two other cancer survivors reveal how they coped with treatment, how they stay well, and what we all should be doing to protect ourselves now.

"You Know Your Body Better Than Anyone"

Cofounder of Oncology Rehab Partners and an assistant professor in the department of physical medicine and rehabilitation at Harvard Medical School, physiatrist Julie K. Silver, MD, was diagnosed with invasive breast cancer in 2003.

"It's nothing. Stop worrying." That was the message Dr. Silver got from her own doctor in 2001, when both a mammogram and ultrasound looked clear. "I was relieved, yet I couldn't shake this uneasy feeling," she says. "I know my breasts, and some tissue in the left one felt subtly different than it used to feel."

To allay her nagging worry, she saw a breast surgeon a few months later. Again the tests turned up normal.

"I should have been totally relieved, but there was this small part of me that continued to worry," she says. "I don't worry excessively about my health, so this was very unusual." Still, she was embarrassed to call the breast surgeon again. "But I had three kids under the age of 12, so I knew I had to risk humiliation and get this looked at one more time," she says.

After the third mammogram, the empathetic surgeon returned to the exam room with tears in her eyes. "She said, 'I'm so sorry. You were right.' It was the most awful moment. I was consumed with emotions—sadness, grief, fear."

Because the diagnosis took 2 years, the cancer was no longer in the earliest stage. "But my oncologist said I had an 'overwhelmingly positive prognosis' because the cancer wasn't terribly aggressive. That phrase became my mantra." Dr. Silver was also armed with hopeful statistics. "There are 11 million cancer survivors in this country—and lots of them were diagnosed after the cancer had spread beyond the breast," she says. "Even with fairly advanced cancer, you can still live a long, reasonably healthy life."

HER STAY-HEALTHY ADVICE

Treat yourself like a cherished friend: "That means giving yourself a break when you need it. Your physical health and emotional health are intertwined. It's important to pay attention to both."

Aim to eat five to nine servings of fruits and vegetables every day: "There is lots of evidence that antioxidants and phytochemicals can keep you healthier overall and may help prevent certain cancers."

"Share Your Experience with Your Family"

Deputy director of the Vanderbilt-Ingram Cancer Center in Nashville and past president of the American Society of Clinical Oncology, David Johnson, MD, was diagnosed with lymphoma in 1989.

When Dr. Johnson discovered lumpy

The Diabetes-Cancer Connection

Yes, there is a connection between diabetes and cancer. For example, overweight or insulin-resistant women are 50 percent more likely to be diagnosed with advanced-stage breast cancer, according to a 20-year study of more than 60,000 Swedish women.

In the study, published in 2008 in the journal *Breast Cancer Research and Treatment*, researchers theorize that hormones linked with overweight or insulin resistance might cause tumors to grow faster.

Additional studies are needed to confirm the connection.

nodes in his groin, he didn't bring it to his doctor's attention for 3 months. "The idea of lymphoma crossed my mind, but I dismissed it. I was 41 and otherwise very healthy," he says.

Not surprisingly, Dr. Johnson was shocked when his doctor told him the results of his biopsy. "My first thought was that I wouldn't live to see my 10-year-old daughter grow up," he says. "Then I started worrying about how she and my wife would survive financially."

Dr. Johnson didn't share those fears with his family, though, which was a lapse he now regrets. "I told my wife I was going to be okay, and after that I didn't talk much about my illness at home. I thought discussing the what-ifs would make her and my daughter anxious, but I think my silence actually made them more nervous," he says. "Now I warn patients that it's important for the family to keep the lines of communication open."

If Dr. Johnson was mum at home, he didn't have that option at work. "I got lots of unsolicited advice from my colleagues, which was nice but often conflicting and confusing," he says. Feeling overwhelmed, he decided not to take too much control of his treatment. "Medical oncologists study for 12 years before they can practice, so it makes sense to trust their judgment," he continues. "I told my doctor that I wanted to get through the treatment as quickly as possible; but aside from that, I left the medical choices up to him."

Now 20 years cancer free, Dr. Johnson is pragmatic about his risk of recurrence: "I take good care of myself, and I try to enjoy everything I can about life."

HIS STAY-HEALTHY ADVICE

Have unusual symptoms checked out ASAP: "If you convey concern when you call your doctor—saying something like 'I'm really worried about this'—then you can usually get an appointment fairly quickly, which can ease your mind."

Sneak in exercise whenever you can: "I always try to use the stairs rather than the elevator, and I walk several mornings a week."

"Embrace Your New Normal"

Dr. Runowicz, who is also a Farmington, Connecticut–based oncologist and past president of the American Cancer Society, was diagnosed in 1992 with breast cancer that had spread to her lymph nodes.

Hearing the words "You have cancer" is terrifying, she says. Hearing that the cancer has spread outside the breast makes you feel doomed. "At first I thought, *I'm dead,*" Dr. Runowicz says. But knowing how important it was to have hope, she reminded herself how effective cancer treatments could be: "I told myself that you didn't have to die from breast cancer."

Her faith in medicine was well founded: After 8 months of chemotherapy, 6 weeks of radiation, and 5 years of tamoxifen, she's been cancer free for 16 years. Although her treatment was grueling—"harder than I expected"—the biggest surprise came after it was over.

"It was like the umbilical cord was cut," she says. "During treatment, you're seeing your doctor every week. Then suddenly you're on your own. You're better, but you're not well. It's hard to know what you're supposed to do next."

To help figure that out, Dr. Runowicz jotted down her thoughts, which eventually became a book, *To Be Alive: A Woman's Guide to a Full Life after Cancer.*

"Writing about my experience helped me regain my footing," she says. Dr. Runowicz also made a radical shift in her health-related habits. "Before cancer, I subsisted on coffee, nervous energy, and whatever looked good in the hospital's snack machines, and I almost never exercised," she says. "After treatment, I became religious about my weight, diet, and working out. Now I'm addicted to the extra energy it gives me. Having cancer forced me to completely rethink the way I approach my own health. I no longer take it for granted."

HER STAY-HEALTHY ADVICE

Create a journal: There, you can grieve for the life you had before a major illness or emotional or physical stress.

Maintain a healthy weight: "I've always been slim, but I wanted to stay that way. Excess body fat produces estrogen and may increase the risk of breast cancer."

Eat a Mediterranean diet: Many studies show a strong link between eating fruits, vegetables, nuts, and olive oil and living longer.

DIABETES

COOKBOOK

THE RECIPES

For this diabetes cookbook, we selected 100 of the very best of this year's *Prevention* recipes. But we were careful to choose recipes with less than 40 percent of their calories from carbohydrates. These recipes are healthy, and they all taste great, too.

Note that recipe analyses—and therefore the carb counts—don't include ingredients that are marked as "optional" or serving suggestions, such as "Try this dish over rice." Take those additional foods into account when counting your carbs.

BREAKFASTS

CHINESE EGG PANCAKES

MAKES 4 SERVINGS

- 2 cups thinly sliced brussels sprouts (about 8 ounces)
- ³/₄ cup thinly sliced scallions (10–12 thin)
- ³/₄ cup shredded carrots
- ¹/₄ teaspoon salt
- 4 large eggs
- 2 large egg whites
- 1 tablespoon grated fresh ginger
- 2 tablespoons water
- 6 teaspoons ground flaxseed

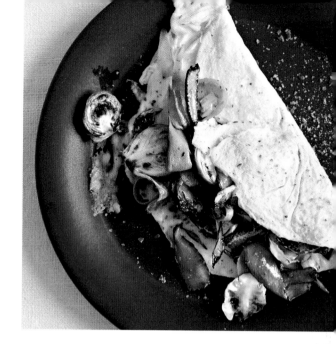

1. Coat a large nonstick skillet with cooking spray. Add the brussels sprouts, scallions, carrots, and salt. Toss to mix. Cover and cook over medium heat, tossing occasionally, for 7 to 10 minutes, or until the vegetables are wilted and lightly browned. Reduce the heat slightly if the vegetables are browning too fast.
2. Meanwhile, beat the eggs, egg whites, ginger, and water with a fork in a mixing bowl.
3. Heat a 9″ nonstick omelet pan over medium-high heat. Turn off the heat and coat the surface with cooking spray. Turn the heat back on, to medium. Ladle one-quarter of the egg mixture (5 tablespoonfuls) into the pan. Cook for 20 to 30 seconds, or until the edges start to set. Using a silicone spatula, carefully lift the edges, tipping the pan to allow runny mixture to get underneath. When the eggs are almost set and just shimmering on top, about 1 minute, sprinkle on 1¹/₂ teaspoons flaxseed and ¹/₂ cup of the vegetable mixture. Cook for about 30 seconds, or until the eggs are completely set.
4. Slide the pancake onto a dinner plate, or roll the pancake like a jelly roll before sliding onto the plate.
5. Repeat for the remaining 3 pancakes.

Note: *To prepare 1 large pancake instead of 4 individual ones, after the vegetables are wilted in step 1, remove them to a plate. Wipe the skillet with a paper towel. Continue with the recipe, using the large skillet instead of the 9″ omelet pan and adding all the ingredients at once. Cooking time will increase slightly. To serve, cut into 4 wedges or slide the whole pancake onto a work surface, roll like a jelly roll, and cut into 4 spirals.*

PER SERVING:

140 CAL

11 g protein	
11 g carbohydrates	
4 g fiber	
6 g fat	
1 g saturated fat	
180 mg cholesterol	
273 mg sodium	

BREAKFAST EGGS

PER SERVING:
159 CAL

18 g protein

3 g
carbohydrates

0 g fiber

8 g fat

3 g
saturated fat

15 mg
cholesterol

510 mg sodium

MAKES 1 SERVING

1/2 cup egg substitute

Salt

Ground black pepper

2 tablespoons light cream cheese, cut into small pieces

1. Mix the egg substitute with salt and pepper to taste.
2. Coat a small nonstick skillet with olive oil spray and heat over medium-low heat. Pour the seasoned egg substitute into the skillet and cook, stirring a few times, until almost set. Gently fold in the cream cheese. Cook for 1 minute longer. Remove the skillet from the heat, cover, and let stand until the cream cheese has melted.

EGG SANDWICH

PER SERVING:
381 CAL

23 g protein

35 g
carbohydrates

9 g fiber

19 g fat

6 g
saturated fat

227 mg
cholesterol

617 mg sodium

MAKES 1 SANDWICH

1 whole egg

1 egg white

1/4 cup mashed Hass avocado

1 whole wheat English muffin, toasted

1 slice reduced-fat Cheddar cheese

Tomato slices

1. Coat a skillet with cooking spray. Scramble the egg with the egg white in the skillet.
2. Spread the avocado on the English muffin. Place the egg on the bottom half of the muffin and top with the cheese, tomato, and other half of the muffin.

FRITTATA

MAKES 4 SERVINGS

6 large eggs

½ cup freshly grated Parmesan cheese

½ teaspoon salt

¼ teaspoon freshly ground black pepper

2 tablespoons olive oil

1 onion, chopped

2 tablespoons chopped parsley (optional)

PER SERVING:

217 CAL

13 g protein
3 g carbohydrates
0.5 g fiber
17 g fat
5 g saturated fat
326 mg cholesterol
550 mg sodium

1. Preheat the oven to 400°F.
2. Whisk the eggs, cheese, salt, and pepper in a medium bowl until just combined. Set aside.
3. Heat the oil in a medium ovenproof nonstick skillet over medium heat. Add the onion and cook for about 5 minutes, or until just browned. Pour the eggs into the skillet and reduce the heat to low. Cook for about 7 minutes, or until the frittata is almost done but the top remains runny.
4. Put in the oven and bake for 4 to 6 minutes, or until lightly browned. Loosen with a spatula, slide onto a serving plate, and sprinkle with the parsley, if desired.

Notes: *If the handle of your skillet isn't ovenproof, wrap it in 4 layers of foil to protect it from the heat.*

You could substitute egg whites for 2 or 3 of the whole eggs.

Variation: *Tuck in a few leftovers if you like, or vary it by adding almost any meat, fish, vegetable, cheese, or herb. Serve warm or at room temperature.*

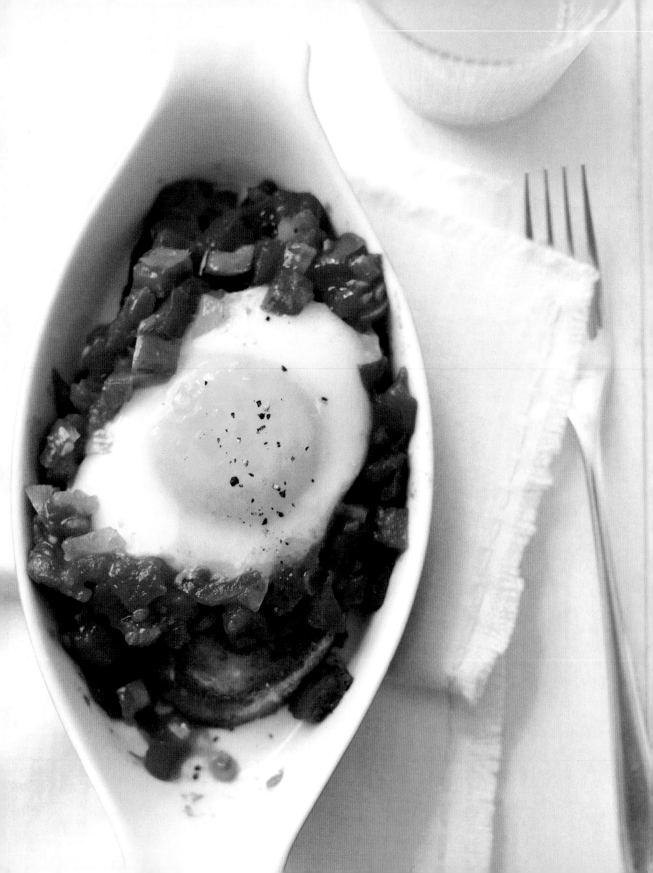

ITALIAN-STYLE EGGS

MAKES 4 SERVINGS

4 slices ($\frac{1}{2}$" thick) French or Italian bread (about 4 ounces)

$\frac{1}{4}$ cup canola oil

$\frac{1}{4}$ cup finely chopped onion

$\frac{1}{4}$ cup finely chopped green bell pepper

6 plum tomatoes, chopped

$\frac{1}{8}$ teaspoon salt

$\frac{1}{8}$ teaspoon ground black pepper

4 large eggs

PER SERVING:

309 CAL

| 11 g protein |
| 23 g carbohydrates |
| 2 g fiber |
| 20 g fat |
| 3 g saturated fat |
| 210 mg cholesterol |
| 350 mg sodium |

1. Heat a large nonstick skillet over medium-high heat. Brush 1 side of each bread slice with some of the oil. Place oil side down in the pan. Brush the tops with the oil. Cook for about 2 minutes on each side, or until toasted. Place a slice of toast on each of 4 plates. Set aside.

2. Return the pan to medium heat. Add the remaining oil and the onion and bell pepper. Cook, stirring, for 2 minutes, or until the vegetables have softened. Stir in the tomatoes, salt, and black pepper. Bring to a boil. Reduce the heat to medium-low and cook for 5 minutes, or until the tomatoes make a chunky sauce. With a large spoon, create 4 indentations in the sauce.

3. Break 2 of the eggs into 2 custard cups. Gently tip each egg into 1 of the indentations in the sauce. Repeat with the remaining 2 eggs. Cover and simmer for 6 to 8 minutes, or until the whites are completely set.

4. Use a large spoon to lift each egg and accompanying sauce onto each plate, either next to or on top of the toast. Spoon any remaining sauce evenly around the egg.

SCRAMBLED EGG "PIZZA"

PER SERVING:
232 CAL

8 g protein	
6 g carbohydrates	
1 g fiber	
19 g fat	
4 g saturated fat	
210 mg cholesterol	
230 mg sodium	

MAKES 4 SERVINGS

- 4 large eggs
- 2 large egg whites
- $\frac{1}{8}$ teaspoon salt
- $\frac{1}{8}$ teaspoon ground black pepper
- 1 whole wheat tortilla (8" diameter)
- $\frac{1}{4}$ cup olive oil
- 1 tomato, chopped
- $\frac{1}{2}$ teaspoon dried oregano
- 1 tablespoon shredded reduced-fat Italian cheese blend

1. Beat the eggs, egg whites, salt, and pepper in a bowl. Set aside.
2. Brush both sides of the tortilla with some of the oil. Heat a nonstick skillet (large enough to hold the tortilla) over medium heat. Place the tortilla in the skillet and cook for about 1 minute, or until golden. Turn with tongs and cook for about 1 minute, or until crisp. Place on a cutting board or platter.
3. Return the skillet to the heat. Add two-thirds of the remaining oil. Swirl to coat the pan. Add the reserved eggs. Stir with a silicone spatula and cook for about 2 minutes, or until set. Spoon evenly over the tortilla.
4. Return the pan to the heat. Add the remaining oil. Swirl to coat the pan. Add the tomato and oregano. Toss for 2 minutes, or until the tomato starts to get juicy. Spoon evenly over the eggs. Sprinkle with the cheese. Cut into 4 wedges with a pizza cutter and serve.

AVOCADO BREAKFAST MUFFIN

MAKES 1 SERVING

¼ ripe avocado, mashed

1 whole wheat or multigrain English muffin, split and toasted

1 egg

1 slice Canadian bacon or extra-thin sliced deli ham

½ slice reduced-fat Colby–Monterey Jack cheese

PER SERVING:

328 CAL

22 g protein

30 g carbohydrates

6 g fiber

15 g fat

3.5 g saturated fat

229 mg cholesterol

801 mg sodium

1. Spread the avocado over the bottom half of the muffin. Place on a plate and set aside.
2. Coat a small nonstick skillet with butter-flavored cooking spray and heat over medium heat. Crack the egg into the skillet and cook until the egg white is solid. Gently slide a spatula under the egg to break the yolk, using the spatula to keep the yolk beneath the white.
3. Place the bacon and cheese over the egg and cook for 2 minutes, or until the cheese melts. Slide the egg mixture onto the muffin with the avocado. Top with the remaining muffin half.

PEANUT BUTTER AND JELLY "PANCAKE"

PER SERVING:

326 CAL

10 g protein	
26 g carbohydrates	
4 g fiber	
20 g fat	
3 g saturated fat	
16 mg cholesterol	
307 mg sodium	

MAKES 1 SERVING

1 frozen homemade or store-bought whole wheat pancake

1 teaspoon honey

¼ teaspoon cornstarch

¼ cup fresh or frozen and thawed blueberries

2 tablespoons peanut butter

1. Heat the pancake in a toaster oven to the desired crispness.
2. Combine the honey and cornstarch in a microwaveable bowl until smooth. Stir in the blueberries. Microwave on high power for 90 seconds, or until bubbling and thickened.
3. Spread the peanut butter on the pancake. Add the fruit mixture.

OAT GRIDDLE CAKES WITH MELTED CHEDDAR

MAKES 4 SERVINGS (2 CAKES EACH)

- 1/4 cup + 2 tablespoons regular oats
- 1/4 cup white whole wheat flour (such as King Arthur)
- 2 tablespoons nonfat dry milk
- 1 tablespoon ground flaxseed
- 1/2 teaspoon baking soda
- 1/2 teaspoon baking powder
- 1/4 teaspoon ground nutmeg
- Pinch of salt
- 1 large egg
- 3 tablespoons low-fat plain yogurt
- 1 1/2 tablespoons canola oil
- 1/4 cup shredded reduced-fat Cheddar cheese

PER SERVING:

165 CAL

7 g protein
14 g carbohydrates
2 g fiber
9 g fat
2 g saturated fat
51 mg cholesterol
376 mg sodium

1. Combine the oats, flour, dry milk, flaxseed, baking soda, baking powder, nutmeg, and salt in a bowl. Stir to mix well.

2. Beat the egg with a fork in a small bowl. Add the yogurt and oil. Whisk with a fork to blend. Add to the dry ingredients and stir just until mixed. Set aside for 5 minutes.

3. Set a griddle or nonstick skillet over medium-high heat for 1 minute. Turn off the heat and coat the griddle or skillet with cooking spray. Turn the heat back on. Dollop the batter in 8 portions onto the griddle or skillet. Cook for about 2 minutes, or until the griddle cakes are browned on the bottom. Flip and press down with the back of a pancake turner to flatten each into a 1/2"-thick disk. Cook for 2 to 3 minutes, or until cooked through. Turn off the heat. Sprinkle the cheese on the oat cakes. Cover with a lid or sheet of aluminum foil. Allow to sit for 2 minutes, or until the cheese melts.

Make it ahead: *Because your time is worth money, it pays to double this recipe and freeze the extras. You'll have nutritious breakfast fare in the freezer without convenience-food prices. Cool the cakes and lay them on a tray. Place in the freezer for 24 hours, or until frozen solid. Pack into zip-top freezer bags. To serve, remove the number you need and thaw at room temperature or in the microwave. Place on a piece of aluminum foil. Top each cake with cheese. Place in a toaster oven for 1 minute, or until the cheese melts.*

SWEET LEMON-RICOTTA BRUNCH BLINTZES

PER SERVING:
308 CAL

| 17 g protein |
| 33 g carbohydrates |
| 5 g fiber |
| 12 g fat |
| 4 g saturated fat |
| 111 mg cholesterol |
| 181 mg sodium |

MAKES 4 SERVINGS (2 BLINTZES EACH)

BLINTZES

- ³/₄ cup white whole wheat flour (such as King Arthur)
- 2 tablespoons ground flaxseed
- Pinch of salt
- 2 large eggs
- 1 tablespoon canola oil
- 1 teaspoon vanilla extract
- 1–1¹/₄ cups fat-free milk

FILLING

- 1 cup part-skim ricotta
- 2 tablespoons confectioners' sugar, plus extra for garnish
- ¹/₄ teaspoon lemon extract
- 1 cup fresh or frozen and thawed raspberries

1. **To make the blintzes:** Combine the flour, flaxseed, and salt in a mixing bowl. Stir to mix.
2. Beat the eggs with a fork or whisk in another mixing bowl until very well blended. Add the oil, vanilla extract, and 1 cup of the milk. Whisk to mix. Add gradually to the dry ingredients, whisking constantly, to create a smooth batter. Allow to sit for 5 minutes.
3. Stir the batter gently and let it run off of a spoon. It should be thinner than cake batter. Add 1 tablespoon more milk at a time until the desired consistency is reached.
4. Heat a crepe pan or 8″ nonstick skillet over medium-high heat. Pick up the pan with a mitt and, holding it away from the heat, coat the pan lightly with cooking spray. Return to medium-high heat. Ladle a scant ¹/₄ cup batter into the pan. Swirl the pan quickly and evenly to cover the bottom with batter. Cook for 1 to 2 minutes, adjusting the heat higher or lower as needed, or until the bottom is browned. Flip and cook for 1 to 2 minutes, or until cooked through. Reduce the heat if the bottoms are browning too fast. Transfer to a tray. Off the heat, coat the pan with cooking spray. Return to the heat and cook another blintz. Continue until all of the blintzes are cooked.

1. **To make the filling:** Preheat the oven to 350°F. Coat a 13″ × 9″ baking dish with cooking spray.
2. Combine the ricotta, sugar, and lemon extract in a bowl. Set aside.
3. Lay the blintzes on a work surface. Dollop some of the ricotta mixture in the center of each blintz. One at a time, fold 2 opposite sides of a blintz over the cheese to meet in the middle. Fold the opposite sides to the middle to make a bundle. Place seam side down in the baking dish. Continue until all of the bundles are shaped. Cover the pan tightly with aluminum foil.
4. Bake for 25 to 30 minutes, or until heated through. Serve warm, garnished with the raspberries and dusted with sugar.

Make it ahead: *If you want, you can make your blintzes several days or even weeks in advance of when you need them. Cool them and stack between small sheets of waxed paper, then place in an airtight container or resealable plastic bag. Refrigerate for up to 3 days or freeze for up to 3 weeks. Allow to thaw before filling and baking.*

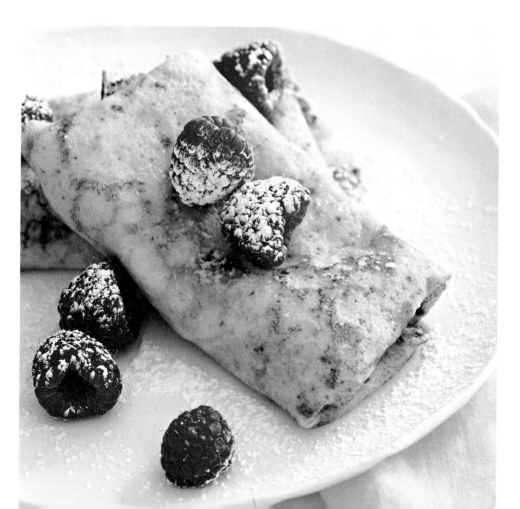

APPETIZERS AND SNACKS

PECAN-CRUSTED CHICKEN TENDERS WITH PEACH SAUCE

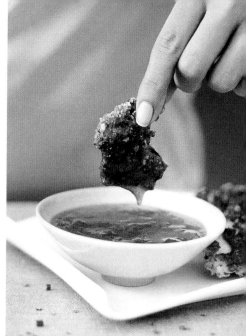

MAKES 4 SERVINGS

- $1/2$ cup pecan halves
- 2 slices whole wheat bread, torn into pieces
- 2 egg whites, lightly beaten
- 1 pound chicken breast tenders (cut if necessary to equal 12 pieces total)
- 1 teaspoon finely chopped fresh thyme or $1/4$ teaspoon dried
- $1/4$ teaspoon salt
- $1/4$ teaspoon freshly ground black pepper
- 1 tablespoon + 1 teaspoon olive oil
- $1/2$ cup apricot or peach 100% fruit spread
- 2 tablespoons freshly squeezed lemon juice (from 1 lemon)

1. Preheat the oven to 425°F. Coat a rimmed baking sheet with cooking spray.
2. Put the pecans in a food processor and chop. Add the bread and pulse to fine crumbs. Transfer to a shallow dish.
3. Put the egg whites in another dish and beat lightly. Sprinkle the chicken with the thyme, salt, and pepper.
4. Dip a piece of chicken into the egg whites and then roll in the crumbs, pressing to adhere. Place on the prepared baking sheet. Repeat with the remaining chicken. Drizzle the chicken with the oil. Bake for 12 to 15 minutes, or until the crumbs brown and the chicken is no longer pink in the thickest part.
5. Mix the fruit spread and lemon juice in a bowl to make a sauce.

PER SERVING (3 TENDERS WITH 2 TABLESPOONS SAUCE):

381 CAL

28 g protein	
29 g carbohydrates	
2 g fiber	
18 g fat	
3 g saturated fat	
63 mg cholesterol	
294 mg sodium	

SWEDISH NUTS

PER SERVING:
168 CAL

5 g protein	
8 g carbohydrates	
3 g fiber	
14 g fat	
2 g saturated fat	
0 mg cholesterol	
9 mg sodium	

MAKES 10 SERVINGS

- 1 egg white
- 1 tablespoon water
- 2 cups mixed plain nuts (pecans, walnuts, and almonds)
- 2 tablespoons Splenda
- 2 teaspoons ground cinnamon
- 1/2 teaspoon pure vanilla extract

1. Preheat the oven to 350°F. Coat a large shallow baking sheet with cooking spray.
2. Beat the egg white and water with a fork in a bowl. Add the nuts. Toss to coat thoroughly with the egg mixture. Place on the baking sheet.
3. Combine the Splenda and cinnamon in a small bowl. Stir to mix. Sprinkle the mixture over the nuts. Drizzle with the vanilla extract. Toss the nuts to coat evenly with the Splenda mixture. Spread the nuts out in a single layer.
4. Bake, stirring occasionally, for 25 to 30 minutes, or until toasted.

GARLIC-CHILI POPCORN

MAKES 10 SERVINGS

2 tablespoons extra-virgin olive oil

1 clove garlic, minced

1 teaspoon red-pepper flakes

10 cups freshly air-popped popcorn (about $1/2$ cup dry)

Pinch of salt

1. In a small skillet, combine the oil, garlic, and pepper flakes. Cook over medium-low heat for about 2 minutes, or until the garlic is soft and the mixture is aromatic. Cool for 5 minutes.

2. Place the popcorn in a large bowl. Pour the oil mixture over the popcorn. Add the salt and toss to coat. Serve immediately.

PER SERVING:

57 CAL

1 g protein

6 g carbohydrates

1 g fiber

3 g fat

<1 g saturated fat

0 mg cholesterol

16 mg sodium

FROM-THE-PANTRY SALSA

MAKES 4 SERVINGS

1 cup drained canned diced tomatoes

$1^1/2$ teaspoons white wine or cider vinegar

1 teaspoon olive oil

1 teaspoon finely chopped cilantro, parsley, or freeze-dried chives

$1/4$ teaspoon garlic powder

8–10 drops hot-pepper sauce

Salt

Combine the tomatoes, vinegar, oil, herb, garlic powder, and hot-pepper sauce and season with salt to taste.

PER SERVING:

23 CAL

1 g protein

2 g carbohydrates

0.5 g fiber

1 g fat

0.5 g saturated fat

TK mg cholesterol

153 mg sodium

Note: *Serve this easy salsa with your favorite veggies or chips.*

"FRIED" ZUCCHINI STICKS WITH MARINARA SAUCE

PER SERVING
(4 STICKS
WITH 2
TABLESPOONS
SAUCE):

219 CAL

6 g protein

14 g
carbohydrates

2 g fiber

16 g fat

2.5 g
saturated fat

3 mg
cholesterol

401 mg sodium

MAKES 4 SERVINGS

- ¼ cup olive oil
- 2 large egg whites
- ¾ cup plain trans-free panko bread crumbs
- 3 tablespoons grated Parmesan cheese
- ¾ teaspoon salt-free Italian herb seasoning
- ¼ teaspoon salt
- 2 medium zucchini (about 12 ounces total), halved crosswise and then cut lengthwise into 1" wedges (16 total)
- ½ cup marinara sauce, warmed

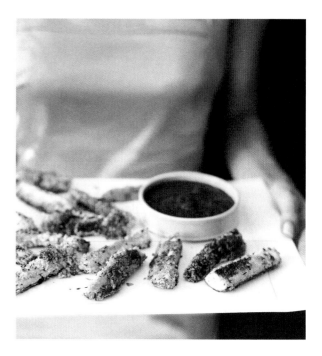

1. Preheat the oven to 425°F. Brush a 17" × 14" jelly roll pan with 1 tablespoon of the oil. (Or use 2 smaller rimmed baking sheets, brushing each with ¹/₂ table-spoon of the oil, and switch the positions of the pans halfway through baking.)
2. Put the egg whites in a shallow dish and beat lightly. Mix the panko, cheese, Italian seasoning, and salt in another shallow dish.
3. Dip the zucchini in the egg whites, one at a time, letting the excess drip off. Roll in the crumbs, pressing them so they adhere. Arrange close together but not touching on the prepared pan. Drizzle with the remaining 3 tablespoons oil.
4. Bake without turning for 25 to 30 minutes, or until the zucchini are crisp and golden. Serve with the marinara sauce for dipping.

Note: *Panko are Japanese bread crumbs that give an irresistible crunch. Avoid brands that contain partially hydrogenated oils (trans fat); we like Ian's.*

BLACK OLIVE TOASTS

MAKES 4 SERVINGS

4 thin slices bread

½ cup drained pitted kalamata olives

1 scallion, sliced

1 teaspoon olive oil

1. Spray the bread with olive oil and toast until golden.
2. Pulse the olives, scallion, and oil in a small food processor or chopper until the mixture comes together.
3. Spread the olive mixture on the toast. Cut each slice in half on the diagonal.

PER SERVING:

123 CAL

2 g protein

12 g
carbohydrates

1 g fiber

7.5 g fat

1 g
saturated fat

0 mg
cholesterol

455 mg sodium

PESTO PINWHEELS

PER SERVING:

185 CAL

12 g protein
9 g carbohydrates
2 g fiber
12 g fat
3 g saturated fat
320 mg cholesterol
350 mg sodium

MAKES 4 SERVINGS (2 SLICES EACH)

- 3 cups baby spinach
- 2 tablespoons all-purpose flour
- 1/4 cup water
- 4 large eggs
- 2 large egg yolks
- 1/8 teaspoon salt
- 1/8 teaspoon ground black pepper
- 1/8 teaspoon paprika
- 1/2 cup fat-free small curd cottage cheese
- 1/4 cup pesto sauce
- 8 cherry tomatoes, quartered

1. Wash the spinach and place in a saucepan with any water clinging to its leaves. Cover and cook, tossing, for about 3 minutes, or until wilted. Drain and rinse with cold water. Squeeze dry and set aside.
2. Preheat the oven to 350°F. Coat a glass or ceramic 13″ × 9″ baking dish with cooking spray. Set aside.
3. Place the flour in a mixing bowl and whisk in the water until smooth. Add the eggs, egg yolks, salt, pepper, and paprika. Beat until smooth. Pour into the baking dish. Bake for 15 minutes, or until firm. Set the egg sheet aside to cool.
4. Process the cottage cheese and reserved spinach in a food processor until smooth. Add the pesto and pulse to mix.
5. Spread the mixture over the egg sheet. Starting at 1 long side, roll the egg sheet into a tube like a jelly roll. Cut crosswise into 8 slices. Serve with the tomatoes on the side.

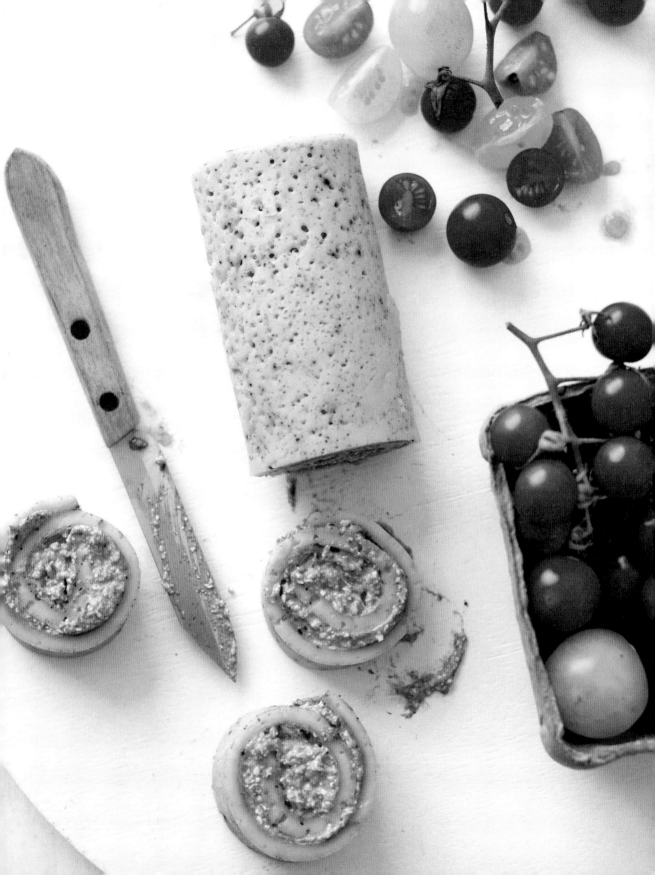

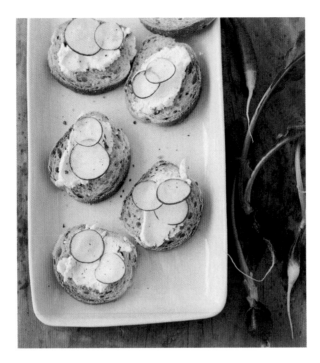

SIMPLE RADISH CANAPÉS

PER SERVING:
125 CAL

3 g protein

7 g
carbohydrates

1 g fiber

10 g fat

7 g
saturated fat

28 mg
cholesterol

214 mg sodium

MAKES 6 SERVINGS

18 slices ($\frac{1}{4}$" each) from small, rustic, whole grain baguette (about 3 ounces)

5 ounces Boursin Garlic & Fine Herbs (see note)

1 bunch radishes (8–12 total), trimmed and sliced into very thin rounds
   Freshly ground black pepper (optional)

1. Spread each slice of bread with $1\frac{1}{2}$ teaspoons Boursin.
2. Layer the radishes on top, overlapping slightly. Season with the pepper, if desired.

Note: *Boursin is a mild cheese that complements the peppery radishes. Extra-thin slices of baguette and radish make these canapés taste better—and easier to eat. Or try crisp flatbread.*

EGGPLANT DIP

MAKES 6 SERVINGS

- 2 large eggplant (about 2 pounds total), halved lengthwise
- 1 large onion (unpeeled), halved
- 3 tablespoons freshly squeezed lemon juice (from 1½ lemons)
- 3 cloves garlic, minced
- 1 tablespoon tahini (sesame paste)
- 1-2 tablespoons water
- ¼ cup olive oil
- 1½ teaspoons salt
- 2 tablespoons chopped parsley

PER SERVING:

138 CAL

2 g protein	
11 g carbohydrates	
5 g fiber	
10.5 g fat	
1.5 g saturated fat	
0 mg cholesterol	
587 mg sodium	

1. Preheat the oven to 425°F. Line a baking sheet with foil and brush with olive oil. Put the eggplant and onion cut side down on the sheet. Bake for about 30 minutes, or until soft and blackened.

2. Remove from the oven and let stand until cool enough to handle. Combine the lemon juice, garlic, and tahini. Stir in the water. Scrape the seeds from the eggplant and discard. Scrape out the remaining flesh, put in a strainer, and press out as much liquid as possible with the back of a spoon. Add to the bowl. Peel and chop the onion. Add to the bowl.

3. Stir in the oil and salt. To serve, drizzle with additional oil, if desired, and sprinkle with the parsley.

WHITE BEAN DIP WITH PISTACHIOS AND CILANTRO

MAKES 6 SERVINGS

1 can (15.5 ounces) cannellini beans, rinsed and drained

1 tablespoon + 1 teaspoon freshly squeezed lemon juice (from $^1/_2$–$^3/_4$ lemon)

1 teaspoon coriander seed, crushed or ground

1 clove garlic, halved

3 tablespoons finely chopped cilantro

3 tablespoons olive oil

3 tablespoons finely chopped pistachios

1 tablespoon finely chopped scallion (white part only)

Salt

Freshly ground black pepper

1. Puree the beans, lemon juice, coriander, and garlic in a food processor until smooth.

2. Stir in the cilantro, oil, pistachios, and scallion. Season the dip to taste with salt and pepper. Transfer to a bowl.

Note: *This dip gets a boost of flavor from cilantro and scallions. Enjoy it on pita wedges, carrot or celery sticks, or bell pepper strips.*

Tip: *Many herbs taste best picked early in the year before flower buds appear. Snip herbs in the morning rather than in the afternoon or evening. The flavorful oils of the plants are most concentrated just after the dew evaporates.*

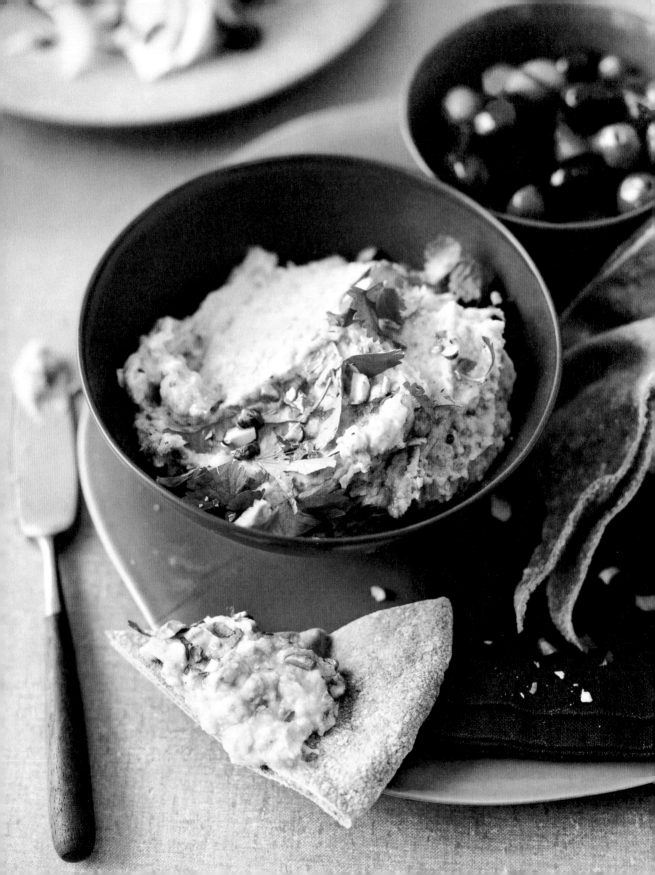

SALADS

ASIAN CUCUMBER SALAD

MAKES 4 SERVINGS

- 3 tablespoons rice wine vinegar
- 2 teaspoons firmly packed dark brown sugar
- 1 tablespoon freshly squeezed lime juice (from $\frac{1}{2}$ lime)
- 1 tablespoon grated fresh ginger
- $\frac{1}{2}$ very small Thai chile pepper, finely chopped, or $\frac{1}{4}$ teaspoon Vietnamese chili paste or $\frac{1}{4}$ teaspoon red-pepper flakes
- 1 tablespoon toasted sesame oil
- 1 large cucumber, peeled and very thinly sliced (2–2$\frac{1}{2}$ cups)
- $\frac{1}{4}$ cup loosely packed, roughly chopped fresh basil
- $\frac{1}{4}$ cup loosely packed, roughly chopped fresh mint
- Salt
- Freshly ground black pepper

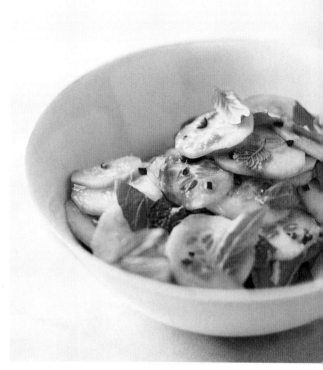

1. Put the vinegar and sugar in a small saucepan and bring to a boil over medium-high heat. Immediately reduce the heat to a steady simmer and cook until reduced to about 1$\frac{1}{2}$ tablespoons. Pour into the serving bowl you're going to use for the salad and let cool for about 10 minutes.
2. Stir in the lime juice; ginger; chile pepper, chili paste, or pepper flakes; and oil.
3. Add the cucumber, basil, and mint and toss until well coated. Taste and adjust seasoning with the salt and black pepper as needed. Serve salad as soon as it's tossed. (You can prepare it ahead, but wait to add the dressing until just before serving.)

Notes: *Be sure to wear plastic gloves when handling fresh or dried chile peppers.*

To turn the salad into a whole meal, add a can of rinsed and drained white beans, a can of drained tuna, and halved cherry tomatoes. You'll need to double the amount of dressing. Serve the main dish salad over lettuce, if you like.

The combination of basil and mint is divine, but if you have only one herb, don't let that keep you from enjoying this fab salad. Simply use double the amount of basil or 1$\frac{1}{2}$ times the quantity of mint suggested.

PER SERVING:
52 CAL
1 g protein

5 g carbohydrates

1 g fiber

4 g fat

0.5 g saturated fat

0 mg cholesterol

5 mg sodium

INSTANT GARDEN SALAD

PER SERVING:

76 CAL

1 g protein
4 g carbohydrates
1 g fiber
7 g fat
1 g saturated fat
0 mg cholesterol
10 mg sodium

MAKES 4 SERVINGS

2 tablespoons olive oil

2 teaspoons freshly squeezed lemon juice (from $^1/_4$-$^1/_2$ lemon)

Salt

Ground black pepper

1 bag (10 ounces) prewashed salad greens

3 scallions, chopped

1. Whisk the oil, lemon juice, and salt and pepper to taste in a large bowl.

2. Add the greens and scallions and toss to coat.

Note: *We like to make this with the multicolored Italian mixed greens that include slightly bitter radicchio balanced by mild romaine and leaf lettuce.*

SPEEDY SPINACH-AND-CARROT SALAD

MAKES 4 SERVINGS

- 1 tablespoon red wine vinegar
- 2 teaspoons firmly packed light brown sugar
- ¼ teaspoon salt
- 3 tablespoons olive oil
- Freshly ground black pepper
- 1 bag (6 ounces) baby spinach
- 2 carrots, grated (1 cup)
- ½ cup dried cranberries (optional)

PER SERVING:

133 CAL

1 g protein

9 g
carbohydrates

3 g fiber

10.5 g fat

1.5 g
saturated fat

0 mg
cholesterol

233 mg sodium

1. Whisk the vinegar, sugar, and salt in a large bowl. Whisk in the oil and season with more salt if needed and the pepper to taste.
2. Add the spinach, carrots, and cranberries (if using), then gently toss to coat. Serve immediately.

Tips: *To make this sweet salad savory, omit the brown sugar and don't add the optional cranberries.*

Homemade dressings are delicious—and easy. Getting salt and sugar to dissolve in oil takes a little effort, but they melt into vinegar almost instantly. So the smart way to stir up a dressing is to start with the vinegar and any ingredients that you want to dissolve, such as salt or mustard, and then add the oil.

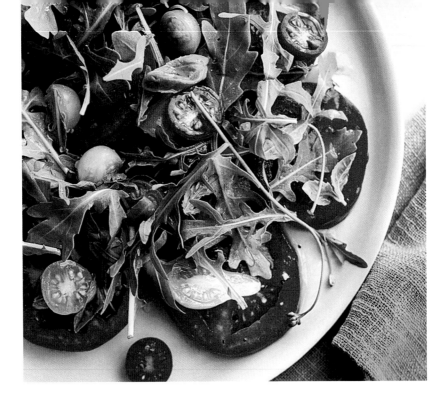

SUMMER TOMATO-AND-ARUGULA SALAD

PER SERVING:

216 CAL

1 g protein	
5 g carbohydrates	
2 g fiber	
21.5 g fat	
3 g saturated fat	
0 mg cholesterol	
10 mg sodium	

MAKES 4 SERVINGS

2 large beefsteak tomatoes, sliced

2 tablespoons red wine, balsamic, or sherry vinegar

$1/8$ teaspoon Dijon mustard (optional)

$1/4$ cup + 2 tablespoons extra-virgin olive oil

Salt

Ground black pepper

2 cups baby arugula or other baby greens

$1/2$ pint yellow and/or red cherry tomatoes, halved

1 cup torn basil leaves or other fresh herb (optional)

1. Arrange the tomato slices on a large platter.
2. Whisk the vinegar and mustard, if using, in a large bowl. Add the oil in a stream while whisking. Season with the salt and pepper to taste.
3. Add the greens and cherry tomatoes to the bowl and toss with the vinaigrette to coat. Spread over the tomato slices. Sprinkle with the basil, if using.

Note: *Two types of tomatoes make an eye-catching salad, but three beefsteaks or a full pint of cherry tomatoes works, too.*

AVOCADO SALAD

MAKES 4 SERVINGS

- 4 very thin slices red onion, separated into rings
- 2 oranges
- 2 avocados
- 3 tablespoons olive oil
- 2 tablespoons chopped fresh mint
- 1 tablespoon freshly squeezed lemon juice (from $\frac{1}{2}$ lemon)
- $\frac{1}{4}$ teaspoon salt

1. Soak the onion in a small bowl of ice water to crisp. Peel the oranges with a knife, removing all of the white pith. Cut crosswise into thin wheels.
2. Pit, peel, and slice the avocados and put in a medium bowl. Drain the onion well and add to the bowl along with the oranges, oil, mint, lemon juice, and salt. Toss to coat.

Notes: *A ripe avocado is just slightly pliant when gently pressed. Avocados ripen at room temperature—faster if you put them in a closed paper bag to capture the ethylene gas (which promotes ripening) given off by the fruit.*

To prevent the browning of a cut avocado, spread the surface with lemon juice, lime juice, or vinegar.

Refrigerate cut avocados in plastic wrap pressed directly onto the cut surface. When ready to eat, scrape off any discoloration; the flavor won't be affected.

PER SERVING:
286 CAL

3 g protein
18 g carbohydrates
9 g fiber
25 g fat
3.5 g saturated fat
0 mg cholesterol
153 mg sodium

GREEN SALAD WITH NUTS AND SEEDS

PER SERVING:
299 CAL

7 g protein
11 g carbohydrates
4 g fiber
27 g fat
4 g saturated fat
9 mg cholesterol
431 mg sodium

MAKES 4 SERVINGS

DRESSING

2 tablespoons freshly squeezed lemon juice (from 1 lemon)

1 tablespoon balsamic vinegar

1 teaspoon prepared mustard

$\frac{1}{2}$ teaspoon salt

2 tablespoons olive oil

1 tablespoon orange juice

$\frac{1}{8}$ teaspoon freshly ground black pepper

SALAD

2 hearts of romaine (9 ounces total), torn into bite-size pieces, about 4 cups

1$\frac{1}{2}$ ounces feta cheese, crumbled

1 cup cherry tomatoes, halved

$\frac{1}{2}$ cup walnut halves, toasted and roughly chopped

$\frac{1}{4}$ cup unsalted, dry-roasted sunflower seeds

$\frac{1}{4}$ cup pine nuts, toasted

1. **To make the dressing:** Combine the lemon juice, vinegar, mustard, and salt in a jar. Cover and shake to dissolve the mustard and salt. Add the oil, orange juice, and pepper. Cover and shake well.

2. **To make the salad:** Combine the romaine, cheese, tomatoes, walnuts, sunflower seeds, and pine nuts in a large bowl. Pour the dressing over the salad and toss gently.

SPRING GREENS WITH CHIVE VINAIGRETTE

MAKES 6 SERVINGS

PER SERVING:
107 CAL

- 3 tablespoons chopped fresh chives
- 1½ tablespoons white wine vinegar
- ½ teaspoon salt
- ¼ teaspoon freshly ground black pepper
- ¼ cup + ½ tablespoon extra-virgin olive oil
- 8 cups lightly packed mixed spring greens, like arugula, mâche, and frisée

Per serving
1 g protein
2 g carbohydrates
2 g fiber
11 g fat
1.5 g saturated fat
0 mg cholesterol
179 mg sodium

1. Combine the chives, vinegar, salt, and pepper in a large bowl. Lightly crush the chives. Whisk in the oil.
2. Toss in the greens. Divide the salad among 6 plates. Sprinkle with additional chives, if desired.

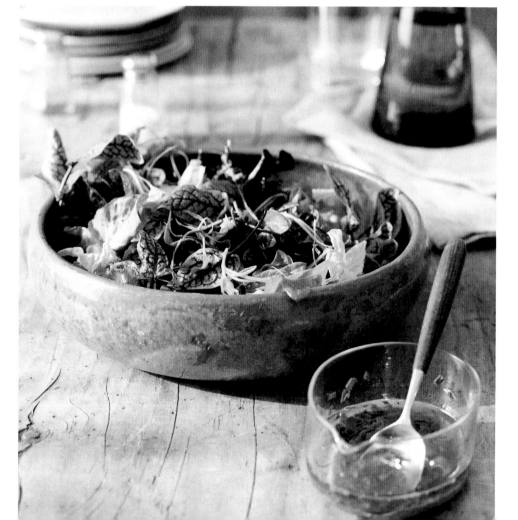

NUT-AND-BERRY SPINACH SALAD

PER SERVING:

218 CAL

3 g protein	
14 g carbohydrates	
4 g fiber	
17 g fat	
2 g saturated fat	
1 mg cholesterol	
62 mg sodium	

MAKES 4 SERVINGS

$\frac{1}{4}$ cup dried blueberries or cranberries

3 tablespoons balsamic vinegar

$\frac{1}{4}$ cup olive oil

Salt

Freshly ground black pepper

1 bag (5–6 ounces) baby spinach

$\frac{1}{4}$ cup slivered or sliced almonds, toasted

1. Combine the berries and vinegar in a salad bowl and let stand for 2 minutes to soften.
2. Whisk in the oil and season with the salt and pepper to taste. Toss with the spinach and almonds.

SHRIMP-AND-CRAB SALAD
WITH EDAMAME AND TARRAGON

MAKES 6 SERVINGS

- 3 tablespoons mayonnaise
- 3 tablespoons sour cream
- 2 tablespoons freshly squeezed lemon juice (from 1 lemon)
- 1/2 teaspoon freshly grated lemon zest
- 1 1/4 pounds chilled cooked shrimp, tails removed
- 12 ounces Dungeness or blue crabmeat
- 1 1/2 cups cooked shelled chilled edamame (soybeans) or frozen edamame, thawed
- 2 scallions (white and green parts), finely chopped
- 1 tablespoon chopped fresh tarragon
- Salt
- Freshly ground black pepper

PER SERVING:
265 CAL
37 g protein

6 g
carbohydrates

1 g fiber

10 g fat

2 g
saturated fat

232 mg
cholesterol

502 mg sodium

1. Whisk the mayonnaise, sour cream, lemon juice, and lemon zest in a large bowl.
2. Add the shrimp, crabmeat, edamame, scallions, and tarragon. Toss gently to coat. Season to taste with the salt and pepper.

Notes: *You can find cooked, shelled edamame (soybeans) in the refrigerator section of most supermarkets. Buy the seafood already cooked, too. If you like, garnish with lemon wedges.*

To keep extra scallions, loosely wrap them in a dry paper towel and put in a zip-top bag. Press out the air and close tightly. Label the bag so it's easy to identify, then store in the crisper drawer. Radishes, carrots, and lettuces keep well this way, too.

BEET-AND-ARUGULA SALAD
WITH SUNFLOWER SEED VINAIGRETTE

PER SERVING:
146 CAL

4 g protein	
6 g carbohydrates	
2 g fiber	
12 g fat	
3 g saturated fat	
7 mg cholesterol	
86 mg sodium	

MAKES 6 SERVINGS

3 medium beets

3 tablespoons olive oil

1 tablespoon red wine vinegar

3 tablespoons unsalted sunflower seeds, toasted

Salt

Freshly ground black pepper

6 cups arugula leaves

2 ounces goat cheese, crumbled ($^1\!/_3$ cup)

1. Preheat the oven to 400°F. Trim the beet stems to about 1″. Wash the beets well. Don't pierce the skin, or they'll bleed.

2. Place the beets on a sheet of foil, fold into an airtight packet, and place on a baking sheet. Bake the beets for about 1 hour, or until tender. When the beets are cool enough to handle, remove the skins and cut the beets into $^1\!/_2$″ cubes. Cover and chill until you're ready to prepare the salad.

3. Whisk the oil, vinegar, seeds, and salt and pepper to taste in a large bowl. Add the arugula, gently toss to coat, and put on salad plates. Arrange the beets and cheese evenly over the top of each salad.

Note: *Naturally sweet beets are lower in calories than they taste. Use red or yellow beets or, for a colorful dish, a mix of both.*

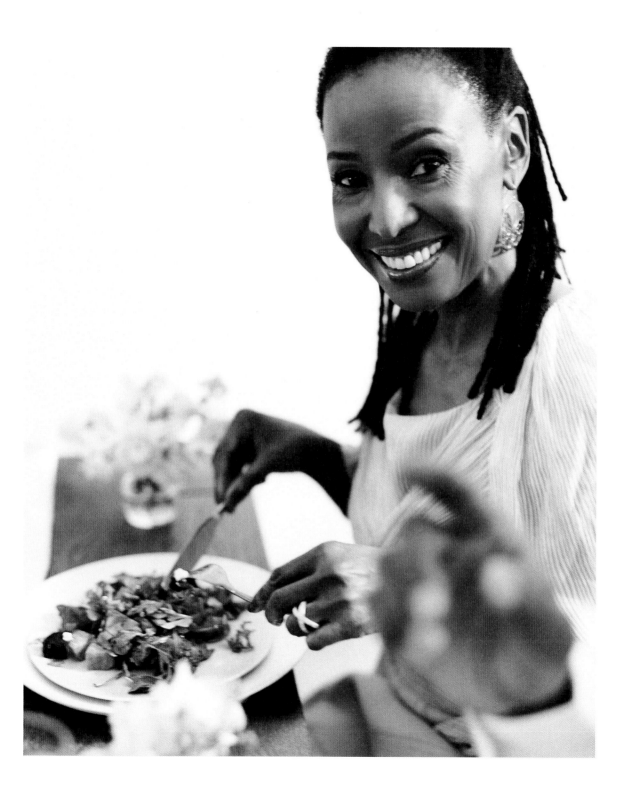

SOUPS

FRENCH ONION SOUP

MAKES 4 SERVINGS (8 CUPS)

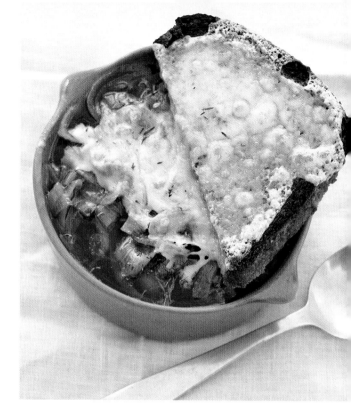

- 2 tablespoons canola oil
- 5 cups sliced onions (about 1¼ pounds)
- 1 teaspoon dried thyme
- 2 bay leaves
- ⅛ teaspoon salt
- ½ cup dry white wine or reduced-sodium vegetable broth
- 4 cups reduced-sodium vegetable broth
- 2 cups water
- 2 slices (1½ ounces each) whole wheat bread, toasted and halved
- 4 teaspoons ground flaxseed
- 6 slices reduced-fat Swiss cheese, halved
  Freshly ground black pepper

1. Preheat the broiler. Heat a pot over medium-high heat. Add the oil and heat for 1 minute. Add the onions, thyme, bay leaves, and salt and stir. Cover and cook, stirring frequently, for about 15 minutes, or until the onions are uniformly browned and softened. Reduce the heat if needed to keep the onions from browning too fast.
2. Add the wine or broth and turn the heat to high. Cook at a brisk simmer for 3 minutes, or until the wine evaporates. Add the 4 cups broth and the water. Bring almost to a boil, then reduce the heat to a simmer. Simmer for 5 minutes. Remove and discard the bay leaves.
3. Place a half slice of toast in the bottom of each of 4 wide, heatproof bowls. Sprinkle 1 teaspoon flaxseed over each toast half. Ladle in the soup. Top each bowlful with 3 half slices of cheese.
4. Broil 6 inches from the heat source for 1 minute, or until the cheese is bubbly and light golden brown. Watch very carefully so the cheese does not burn. Season to taste with the pepper.

PER SERVING:

315 CAL

13 g protein	
28 g carbohydrates	
5 g fiber	
15 g fat	
5 g saturated fat	
20 mg cholesterol	
359 mg sodium	

LEMONY CHICKEN SOUP

PER SERVING:

447 CAL

51 g protein
36 g carbohydrates
6 g fiber
11 g fat
3 g saturated fat
199 mg cholesterol
940 mg sodium

MAKES 4 SERVINGS

- 1 teaspoon olive oil
- 1 small clove garlic, finely chopped
- 6 cups chicken broth (we used Kitchen Basics)
- 1 rib celery, chopped
- 1 cup shredded carrots
- $\frac{1}{2}$ teaspoon freshly ground black pepper
- $\frac{1}{4}$ teaspoon salt
- $\frac{1}{2}$ cup orzo
- $2\frac{1}{2}$ cups frozen green peas or cut-up green beans
- 3 cups chopped cooked chicken (leftover or pulled from a rotisserie chicken)
- 2 large eggs
- 3-4 tablespoons freshly squeezed lemon juice (from 1-2 lemons)

1. Heat the oil in a Dutch oven over medium heat. Add the garlic and cook for about 1 minute, or until lightly browned. Add the broth, celery, carrots, pepper, and salt and bring to a boil over high heat. Add the orzo and reduce the heat to a simmer. Cook for about 8 minutes, or until the orzo is tender.

2. Add the peas or beans and chicken and simmer for 2 minutes.

3. Meanwhile, whisk the eggs and 3 tablespoons of the lemon juice in a medium bowl. Warm the egg mixture gently by whisking in about 1 cup of the hot broth in a thin stream.

4. Whisk the egg mixture into the soup and warm briefly over low heat for 2 minutes. Do not boil or the eggs will curdle. Adjust the seasoning as needed with more lemon juice, salt, or pepper.

Tip: *To extract more lemon juice, before squeezing, warm the whole lemon in the microwave for about 20 seconds or roll it around firmly on a countertop, or both.*

MINI MEATBALL SOUP

MAKES 4 SERVINGS

- 2 teaspoons olive oil
- 8 ounces sliced mushrooms
- 3 cups sliced cabbage
- 1½ teaspoons dried oregano
- 2 cloves garlic, minced
- 2 cups low-sodium beef broth (we used Kitchen Basics)
- 2 cups low-sodium chicken broth (we used Kitchen Basics)
- 2 cups water
- 1 tablespoon tomato paste
- ½ cup rice
- 2 tablespoons fat-free milk
- 6 ounces 80% lean ground beef
- 1 large egg
- ¼ cup grated Parmesan cheese
- 3 tablespoons chopped parsley
- ¾ teaspoon black pepper
- ½ teaspoon salt
- ½ cup roasted red peppers, chopped

PER SERVING:

333 CAL

21 g protein
29 g carbohydrates
3 g fiber
15 g fat
5 g saturated fat
88 mg cholesterol
540 mg sodium

1. Heat the oil in a Dutch oven over medium-high heat. Add the mushrooms and sauté for 4 minutes. Stir in the cabbage, 1 teaspoon of the oregano, and half of the garlic and cook for 1 minute. Add the broths, water, and tomato paste. Reduce the heat to medium.
2. Mix the rice and milk. Add the beef, egg, cheese, 1½ tablespoons of the parsley, black pepper, salt, remaining ½ teaspoon oregano, and remaining garlic. Form mini meatballs, a heaping teaspoon each.
3. Put the meatballs in the broth. Simmer for about 15 minutes, or until the rice in the meatballs is done. Add the red peppers and the remaining 1½ table-spoons parsley. Adjust seasoning with black pepper and salt if needed.

Tip: *Use any kind of ready-sliced mushroom or a combination in this soup.*

Variation: *If you prefer, replace the raw rice with cooked brown rice. White holds the meatballs together better, but they'll taste as good. The simmering time will be the same.*

HOT-AND-SOUR SOUP

PER SERVING:

146 CAL

12 g protein

14 g
carbohydrates

3 g fiber

6 g fat

1 g
saturated fat

45 mg
cholesterol

594 mg sodium

MAKES 4 SERVINGS

4 cups fat-free, reduced-sodium chicken broth

2 teaspoons reduced-sodium soy sauce

$1/8$ teaspoon hot red-pepper sauce

4 ounces shiitake mushrooms, sliced

1 cup snow peas, trimmed and thinly sliced lengthwise

1 carrot, julienned

2 tablespoons grated fresh ginger

3 tablespoons rice wine vinegar

2 tablespoons cornstarch

1 enriched egg, slightly beaten

7 ounces firm tofu with calcium sulfate, drained and cut into $1/4$" cubes

2 scallions, diagonally sliced

1. Heat the broth, soy sauce, and red-pepper sauce in a large saucepan over medium-high heat. Bring to a boil. Add the mushrooms, snow peas, carrot, and ginger. Reduce the heat to low and simmer for 10 minutes, or until the vegetables are tender.

2. Whisk the vinegar and cornstarch in a small bowl. Stir into the soup, then continue to stir for 1 minute, or until thickened. Slowly drizzle the egg into the pan, stirring constantly. Stir in the tofu. Heat gently for another minute. Remove from the heat and let stand, covered, for 1 minute. Top with the scallions.

TURKEY NOODLE SOUP WITH SPINACH

MAKES 8 SERVINGS

PER SERVING:
122 CAL

13 g protein	
12 g carbohydrates	
2 g fiber	
3 g fat	
0 g saturated fat	
17 mg cholesterol	
446 mg sodium	

- 3 ounces whole wheat noodles, cooked
- 1 tablespoon canola oil
- $\frac{1}{2}$ cup chopped onion
- $\frac{1}{2}$ cup chopped carrot
- $\frac{1}{2}$ cup chopped celery
- 1 teaspoon dried sage
- 12 ounces ground turkey breast
- 2 cans ($14\frac{1}{2}$ ounces each) fat-free, reduced-sodium chicken broth
- 4 cups water
- 1 tablespoon balsamic vinegar
- $\frac{1}{2}$ teaspoon salt
- 1 bag (6 ounces) baby spinach
  Freshly ground black pepper

1. Cook the noodles according to the package directions. Drain and set aside.
2. Meanwhile, warm the oil in a pot over medium heat. Add the onion, carrot, celery, and sage. Cook, stirring occasionally, for 5 minutes, or until the vegetables start to soften. Add the turkey. Cook, breaking up the turkey with the back of a spoon, for about 4 minutes longer, or until the turkey is no longer pink.
3. Add the broth, water, vinegar, and salt. Simmer for about 5 minutes, or until hot. Do not boil. Stir in the spinach and reserved noodles. Remove from the heat and let rest for 5 minutes. Season with the pepper to taste.

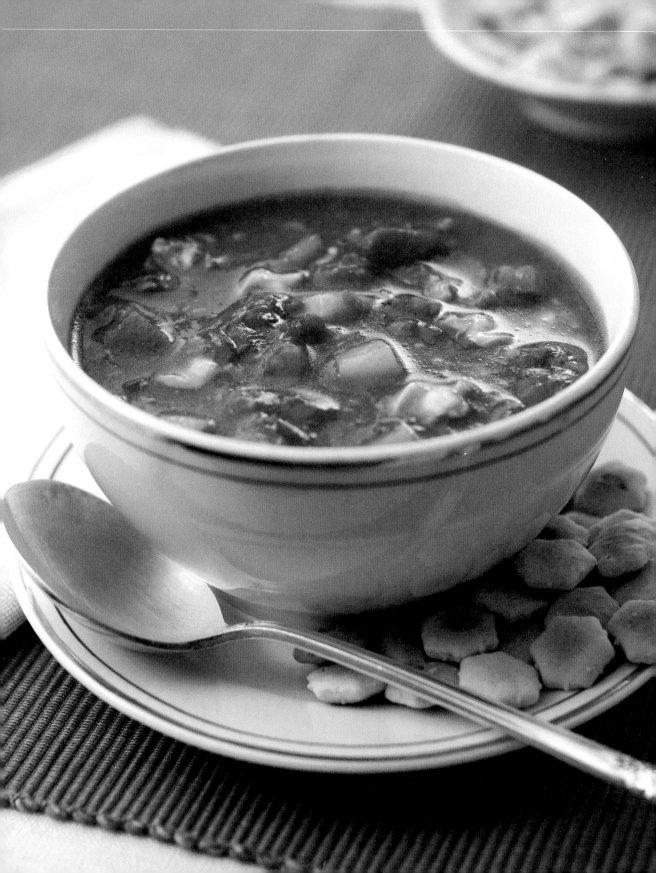

MANHATTAN CLAM CHOWDER

MAKES 6 SERVINGS

PER SERVING:
83 CAL

5 g protein	
8 g carbohydrates	
2 g fiber	
3 g fat	
<1 g saturated fat	
10 mg cholesterol	
388 mg sodium	

- 1 tablespoon canola oil
- 1/2 cup chopped onion
- 1/2 cup chopped bell pepper (any color)
- 1 medium potato, peeled and chopped
- 1/2 cup chopped celery
- 1/2 teaspoon dried thyme
- 1/8 teaspoon paprika
- 1/8 teaspoon salt
- 1 can (14 1/2 ounces) petite diced tomatoes
- 1 tablespoon tomato paste
- 1 can (14 1/2 ounces) vegetable broth or fat-free, reduced-sodium chicken broth
- 1 container (6 ounces) baby clams or littleneck clams, drained

1. Warm the oil in a pot over medium heat. Add the onion, pepper, potato, celery, thyme, paprika, and salt. Cook, stirring, for about 5 minutes, or until the vegetables start to soften.
2. Add the tomatoes, tomato paste, and broth. Simmer for 10 minutes. Add the clams and heat gently just until hot.

CHICKEN-AND-ALMOND DUMPLINGS

MAKES 4 SERVINGS (1 CUP SOUP AND 3 DUMPLINGS EACH)

- 1 tablespoon olive oil
- 3 carrots, cut into 1/2" pieces
- 2 ribs celery, chopped
- 1 onion, finely chopped
- 2 cloves garlic, minced
- 1/2 teaspoon dried thyme
- 3 cups fat-free, reduced-sodium chicken broth
- 1 cup water
- 1 pound boneless, skinless chicken breasts, chopped
- 1/2 cup almonds
- 3/4 cup all-purpose flour
- 1/2 teaspoon baking powder
- 1/4 teaspoon baking soda
- 1/4 teaspoon salt
- 1 tablespoon trans-free margarine
- 6 tablespoons low-fat buttermilk

1. Heat the oil in a large saucepan over medium-high heat. Add the carrots, celery, onion, garlic, and thyme. Cook, stirring occasionally, for 2 to 3 minutes, or until just starting to soften. Stir in the broth and water. Add the chicken. Bring to a boil, reduce to a simmer, cover, and cook for 30 minutes.

2. Meanwhile, bring a large pot of water to a simmer. Place the almonds in a medium skillet and cook over medium-high heat, shaking the pan often, for 3 to 5 minutes, or until lightly toasted. Transfer to a plate to cool for 5 minutes. Place the almonds in a food processor or blender and process to a fine meal.

3. Combine the ground almonds, flour, baking powder, baking soda, and salt in a bowl. With a pastry blender or 2 knives used scissor fashion, cut the margarine into the flour mixture until it resembles coarse crumbs. Stir in the buttermilk until a soft dough forms.

4. Place the dough on a lightly floured surface and pat to a 1/2" thickness. Cut the dough into 12 equal pieces. Drop into the simmering water and cook, turning once, for 17 to 18 minutes, or until the dumplings are cooked through. Remove with a slotted spoon and transfer to the pan with the chicken mixture. Simmer gently for 5 minutes. Divide among 4 bowls.

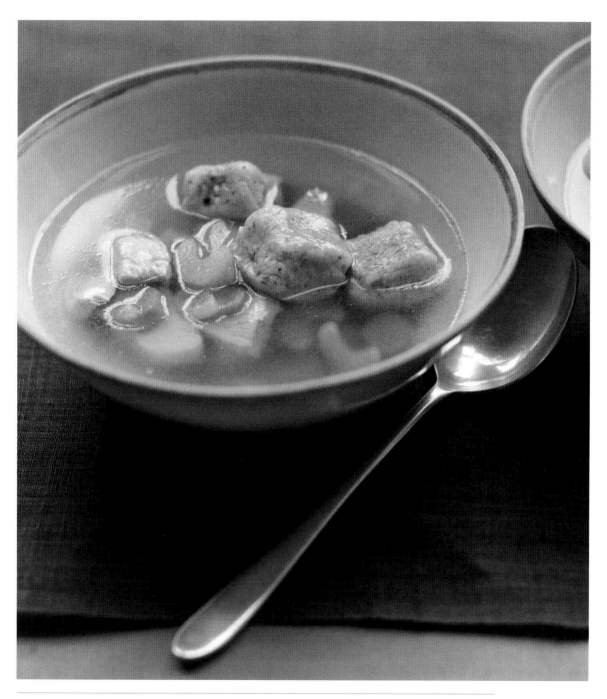

Tip: *For best results, make sure the almonds are finely ground. Nuts provide a nice firmness to the dumplings, but you don't want to detect any little pieces.*

SIDE DISHES

CHILI-BAKED FRIES

MAKES 4 SERVINGS

- ½ teaspoon chili powder
- ¼ teaspoon ground cumin
- ¼ teaspoon dried oregano
- 2 large Yukon gold potatoes, scrubbed, each cut into 10 wedges
- 1 tablespoon canola oil
- ½ cup (2 ounces) shredded low-fat Monterey Jack cheese

1. Preheat the oven to 400°F. Combine the chili powder, cumin, and oregano in a small bowl.
2. Place the potatoes on a baking sheet with sides and sprinkle with the oil and chili powder mixture. Toss to coat. Bake for 40 minutes, turning occasionally, or until tender. Top with the cheese and bake for 2 minutes, or until melted.

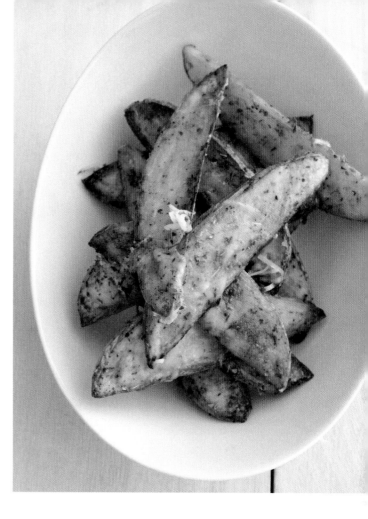

PER SERVING:
141 CAL

6 g protein
16 g carbohydrates
1 g fiber
7 g fat
2 g saturated fat
10 mg cholesterol
127 mg sodium

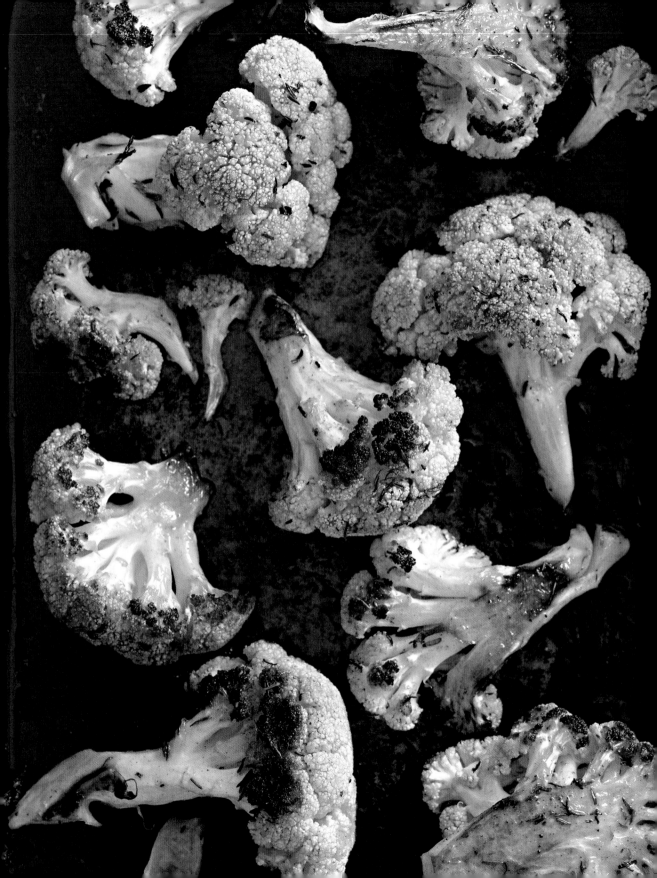

SMOKY CAULIFLOWER

MAKES 4 SERVINGS

1 small head cauliflower, cut into florets

2 tablespoons canola oil

1 teaspoon dried thyme

1/4 teaspoon smoked paprika

1/4 teaspoon salt

1. Preheat the oven to 450°F.
2. Place the cauliflower on a large baking sheet with sides. Drizzle with the oil, thyme, paprika, and salt. Toss to coat. Roast for 20 minutes, turning once, or until browned and tender.

PER SERVING:

79 CAL

1 g protein

4 g carbohydrates

2 g fiber

4 g fat

<1 g saturated fat

0 mg cholesterol

165 mg sodium

SESAME BROCCOLI

PER SERVING:

121 CAL

6 g protein
11 g carbohydrates
3 g fiber
7 g fat
1 g saturated fat
0 mg cholesterol
397 mg sodium

MAKES 4 SERVINGS

6 cups water

1 pound broccoli, cut into florets (about 4 cups)

2 tablespoons reduced-sodium soy sauce

2 teaspoons honey

1 teaspoon rice wine vinegar

1 tablespoon canola oil

1 red onion, cut into wedges

1 clove garlic, minced

4 ounces Asian-style baked tofu, at room temperature, cubed

1 tablespoon sesame seeds

1. Bring the water to a boil in a large stockpot. Add the broccoli and cook for 2 minutes, or until crisp-tender. Drain.

2. Meanwhile, combine the soy sauce, honey, and vinegar in a small bowl. Heat the oil in a large nonstick skillet over medium-high heat. Add the onion and cook, stirring, for 5 minutes, or until lightly browned. Add the broccoli and garlic and cook, stirring, for 3 minutes. Stir the sauce mixture and add to the skillet, stirring for 2 minutes.

3. Sprinkle with the tofu and sesame seeds.

Tip: *Toss any leftover broccoli with mixed greens and fat-free Asian-style salad dressing.*

OLD-FASHIONED CREAMED SPINACH

MAKES 4 SERVINGS

PER SERVING:

142 CAL

11 g protein	
15 g carbohydrates	
6 g fiber	
6 g fat	
2 g saturated fat	
12 mg cholesterol	
432 mg sodium	

3 tablespoons ground flaxseed

1 red onion, chopped

4 ounces mushrooms, sliced

1 clove garlic, minced

$^1/_2$ cup fat-free, reduced-sodium chicken broth

10 ounces baby spinach

3 ounces fat-free cream cheese

$^1/_2$ cup (2 ounces) shredded reduced-fat Cheddar cheese

1 teaspoon Dijon mustard

1. Preheat the oven to 350°F. Coat a $1^1/_2$-quart baking dish with cooking spray and sprinkle the flaxseed over the bottom of the dish.

2. Coat a large nonstick skillet with cooking spray and heat over medium heat. Add the onion and mushrooms and cook, stirring, for 5 minutes, or until tender and the mushrooms have released their juices. Add the garlic and cook, stirring, for 2 minutes, or until lightly browned.

3. Stir in the broth and spinach and cook for 4 minutes, stirring, or until the spinach wilts. Stir in the cheeses and mustard. Stir until just melted and well blended.

4. Pour into a prepared dish. Bake for 20 minutes, or until set. Let stand for 5 minutes before serving.

FAST-AND-FANCY GREEN BEANS

PER SERVING:
73 CAL

3 g protein

8 g
carbohydrates

3 g fiber

4 g fat

0.5 g
saturated fat

0 mg
cholesterol

4 mg sodium

MAKES 8 SERVINGS

- 1 clove garlic, minced or crushed
- 2 teaspoons olive oil
- $\frac{1}{4}$ cup water
- 24 ounces petite (or regular) frozen green beans
- 20 large fresh basil leaves, gently torn
- $\frac{1}{3}$ cup blanched slivered almonds, toasted
- 1 teaspoon cider vinegar
-     Salt
-     Freshly ground black pepper

1. Put the garlic and 1 teaspoon of the oil in a large pot and cook over medium heat for about 2 minutes, or until just beginning to turn golden brown.
2. Add the water and beans, cover, and cook, stirring occasionally, for about 10 minutes, or until heated through.
3. Place 1 cup of the beans in a small food processor along with the basil, almonds, and vinegar. Pulse until the mixture is thoroughly chopped and sticks together. Stir in the remaining 1 teaspoon oil.
4. Stir the pureed mixture into the remaining beans to coat. Season with the salt and pepper to taste.

Tips: *Prepare the pesto like pureed bean sauce up to 3 days ahead, if you like. Cook the rest of the beans and combine them with the sauce a couple of hours before serving.*

This lush veggie tastes as good at room temperature as it does warm—a boon when you're trying to get everything on the table at once.

ROASTED ASPARAGUS
WITH TOASTED WALNUTS

MAKES 4 SERVINGS

PER SERVING:

98 CAL

¼ cup walnuts, chopped

1 pound asparagus, trimmed

1 tablespoon canola oil

1 clove garlic, minced

¼ teaspoon salt

¼ teaspoon freshly ground black pepper

3 g protein

5 g
carbohydrates

2 g fiber

8 g fat

1 g
saturated fat

0 mg
cholesterol

147 mg sodium

1. Preheat the oven to 400°F.
2. Place the walnuts on a large baking sheet with sides and bake for 5 minutes, or until toasted. Place on a plate.
3. Arrange the asparagus in the same baking sheet. Sprinkle with the oil, garlic, salt, and pepper, and then turn to coat.
4. Roast for 12 to 15 minutes, depending on the thickness of the spears, or until lightly browned. Place on a serving plate and sprinkle with the toasted nuts.

ROASTED VEGETABLES

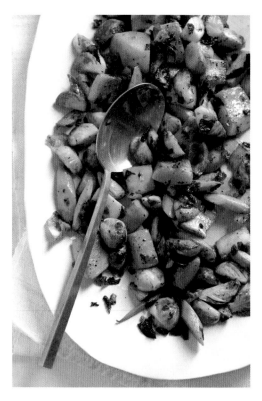

PER SERVING:
171 CAL

3 g protein	
18 g carbohydrates	
6 g fiber	
11 g fat	
1.5 g saturated fat	
0 mg cholesterol	
617 mg sodium	

MAKES 4 SERVINGS

- 1 pound piece of winter squash, such as butternut or acorn, peeled and cut into 1" cubes (2 cups)
- ½ pound brussels sprouts (about 12), quartered
- 3 large carrots, peeled and cut into ¼" diagonal slices
- 1 red onion, chopped
- 3 tablespoons olive oil
- 1 teaspoon salt
- 2 tablespoons chopped fresh parsley
- 1½ tablespoons white wine vinegar
- ¼ teaspoon freshly ground black pepper

1. Preheat the oven to 450°F.
2. Toss the squash, brussels sprouts, carrots, and onion with 2 tablespoons of the oil and ½ teaspoon of the salt in a large bowl. Spread the vegetables in a single layer on a baking sheet (use 2 if necessary) and roast for about 30 minutes, or until browned and tender. Stir once or twice during cooking.
3. Return the vegetables to the bowl and toss with the parsley, vinegar, pepper, and remaining 1 tablespoon oil and ½ teaspoon salt.

Variations: *In spring, try quartered new potatoes and baby beets (segregated at one end of the pan so they don't bleed on the potatoes) and whole asparagus spears. In summer, use sliced red bell pepper and zucchini and cubed eggplant. And in autumn, try halved mushrooms, sliced sweet potatoes or parsnips, and cauliflower florets.*

Tips: *Seeded, peeled, and cut-up butternut squash is available in most supermarkets.*

Judge the cooking time. It varies depending on the type and freshness of the vegetables and the accuracy of your oven, but 25 to 35 minutes is a typical range. Roast until the tip of a paring knife goes in easily. Or simply taste a piece to see whether it's done as you like.

STUFFED ZUCCHINI

MAKES 4 SERVINGS

- 2 large zucchini, halved
- $\frac{1}{4}$ cup olive oil
- 2 medium onions, finely chopped
- 1 pound 95% lean ground beef, lamb, or a combination
- 1 cup cooked rice
- 1 teaspoon ground cinnamon
- 1 teaspoon salt
- $\frac{1}{2}$ teaspoon ground allspice
- $\frac{1}{4}$ teaspoon freshly ground black pepper
  Pinch of red-pepper flakes
- $\frac{1}{4}$ cup pine nuts, toasted
- 1 tablespoon freshly squeezed lemon juice (from $\frac{1}{2}$ lemon), optional
- $\frac{1}{2}$ cup plain yogurt (optional)

PER SERVING:
433 CAL

29 g protein	
24 g carbohydrates	
4 g fiber	
25.5 g fat	
5 g saturated fat	
70 mg cholesterol	
676 mg sodium	

1. Preheat the oven to 350°F.
2. Put the zucchini cut side down on an oiled baking sheet. Bake for 25 minutes. Remove the flesh, leaving $\frac{1}{4}$" of the wall intact. Reserve $\frac{1}{2}$ cup of the flesh.
3. Heat 2 tablespoons of the oil in a skillet over medium-high heat. Add the onions and cook for 10 minutes. Add the beef or lamb and remaining 2 tablespoons oil and cook, breaking up, for 5 to 7 minutes, or until browned.
4. Stir in the rice, cinnamon, salt, allspice, black pepper, pepper flakes, and the reserved zucchini flesh. Cook for 2 to 3 minutes. Stuff the zucchini with the meat filling and top with the nuts.
5. Put the zucchini on the baking sheet and roast for 3 to 5 minutes, or until the filling is lightly browned. Drizzle with the lemon juice and dollop with the yogurt, if desired.

VEGETARIAN MEALS

CONFETTI PESTO PASTA

MAKES 4 SERVINGS

- 1 pint cherry tomatoes
- 1½ cups cooked green beans
- 1½ cups diced chicken breast
- ¼ cup pesto sauce
- ¼ teaspoon salt
- ¼ teaspoon freshly ground black pepper
- 4 cups cooked linguine
- ¼ cup shredded Parmesan cheese

1. Combine the tomatoes, green beans, chicken, pesto, salt, and pepper in a bowl. Add the linguine.
2. Divide among 4 bowls. Garnish with the cheese.

PER SERVING:
346 CAL

27 g protein	
34 g carbohydrates	
2 g fiber	
11 g fat	
4 g saturated fat	
53 mg cholesterol	
392 mg sodium	

SCRAMBLED EGG ENCHILADAS WITH BLACK BEAN SAUCE

MAKES 6 SERVINGS

2 tablespoons vegetable oil

1/2 small onion, sliced 1/4" thick

2 cloves garlic, chopped

1 can (15 ounces) reduced-sodium black beans, with liquid

1 cup water

1 canned chipotle chile pepper in adobo sauce, chopped

1 1/2 teaspoons salt

6 corn tortillas (7"–8" diameter)

4 scallions, thinly sliced

7 large eggs

3 ounces Neufchâtel cheese (reduced-fat cream cheese), cubed

2/3 cup shredded Mexican Chihuahua or Cheddar cheese (about 3 ounces)

2 tablespoons chopped cilantro

1. Preheat the oven to 400°F.
2. Warm 1 tablespoon of the oil in a large skillet over medium heat. Add the onion. Cook for about 7 minutes, or until golden. Add the garlic and cook for 1 minute. Scoop into a blender, leaving the oil. Set the pan aside. Puree with the beans, water, pepper, and 3/4 teaspoon of the salt until smooth. Season with more salt, if desired.
3. Lay the tortillas on a baking sheet. Coat both sides lightly with oil. Stack in twos. Bake for about 3 minutes, or until pliable. Remove, stack, and keep warm.
4. Return the skillet to medium heat. Add the scallions and remaining 1 tablespoon oil. Cook for 2 to 3 minutes, or until soft. Whisk the eggs and remaining 3/4 teaspoon salt. Add to the pan and stir every few seconds until the eggs barely set. Remove from the heat and stir in the cream cheese.
5. Put 1/2 cup of the sauce in an 11" × 7" baking dish. Fill the tortillas with the eggs, roll up, and put in the dish. Pour the rest of the sauce over the enchiladas, completely covering. Sprinkle with the Mexican Chihuahua or Cheddar cheese and bake for 10 to 12 minutes, or until hot. Sprinkle with the cilantro.

Tip: *If desired, you can make the sauce several days before serving. Assemble the enchiladas a couple of hours before warming. Bake for about 15 minutes, or until hot throughout.*

VEGETARIAN CABBAGE "LASAGNA"

MAKES 6 SERVINGS

- 1 head (1½ pounds) green cabbage (about 12 large leaves), cored
- 1 tablespoon olive oil
- ½ cup finely chopped onion (about 1 small)
- 1 pound sliced mushrooms
- 1 bag (6 ounces) baby spinach, cut into slices (about 8 cups loosely packed)
- 1 tablespoon Italian seasoning blend
- 1 package (12–14 ounces) silken tofu, drained
- 2 large eggs, beaten
- ¼ cup (1 ounce) grated Parmesan-Romano cheese blend
- ½ teaspoon ground black pepper
- ¼ teaspoon salt
- ¼ teaspoon ground nutmeg
- 1 jar (26 ounces) marinara sauce
- 1 cup (4 ounces) shredded part-skim mozzarella

PER SERVING:
263 CAL

18 g protein

23 g
carbohydrates

7 g fiber

12 g fat

4 g
saturated fat

88 mg
cholesterol

979 mg sodium

1. Separate the cabbage leaves and wash in cold water. Reserve the remaining cabbage in the refrigerator for another use. Place 4 to 6 leaves in a resealable plastic storage bag. Microwave on high power for 3 to 4 minutes, rotating, or until wilted. Using oven mitts, remove and set aside. Fill another bag with leaves. Microwave until wilted. Empty the first bag; fill it with leaves and microwave. Continue until all the leaves are steamed.

2. Preheat the oven to 350°F. Coat a 13" × 9" pan with cooking spray.

3. Warm the oil in a large nonstick skillet over medium-high heat. Add the onion and mushrooms. Toss to coat. Cover and cook for about 5 minutes, or until the liquid pools in the pan. Uncover and cook for about 4 minutes longer, or until the liquid has evaporated. Add the spinach and seasoning. Cook, stirring, for about 2 minutes, or until the spinach is wilted.

4. Combine the tofu, eggs, Parmesan-Romano, pepper, salt, and nutmeg in a bowl. Stir to blend completely. Coat the bottom of the pan with ¼ cup of the sauce. Line the pan with 4 of the cabbage leaves. Top with half of the tofu mixture, half of the mushroom mixture, and about ⅔ cup sauce. Cover with 4 of the cabbage leaves. Top with the remaining tofu mixture, mushroom mixture, and ⅔ cup sauce. Cover with the remaining leaves and sauce. Sprinkle the mozzarella on top. Bake for about 30 minutes, or until bubbly and the cheese is golden.

SPINACH LASAGNA

PER SERVING:

354 CAL

| 24 g protein |
| 40 g carbohydrates |
| 8 g fiber |
| 13 g fat |
| 6 g saturated fat |
| 35 mg cholesterol |
| 811 mg sodium |

MAKES 8 SERVINGS

1/2 pound whole wheat lasagna noodles (9 or 10 total)

SAUCE

2 teaspoons olive oil

4 cloves garlic, minced

1 can (28 ounces) crushed tomatoes (not in puree)

2 tablespoons tomato paste

3/4 teaspoon dried thyme

1/2 teaspoon dried oregano

1/2 teaspoon salt

1/4 teaspoon freshly ground black pepper

FILLING

2 teaspoons olive oil

1 medium onion, finely chopped

1/2 pound shiitake mushrooms, stemmed and sliced

3 large cloves garlic, minced

2 bunches (1 pound total) spinach, trimmed

1/2 teaspoon salt

1/2 teaspoon freshly ground black pepper

1 container (15 ounces) part-skim ricotta

8 ounces shredded reduced-fat mozzarella

1/3 cup grated Parmesan cheese

1. Preheat the oven to 375°F. Coat a 13" × 9" baking dish with cooking spray.
2. Cook the noodles in boiling salted water for 5 to 8 minutes, or until just done. Drain and rinse under cold water. Lay the noodles on a baking sheet in 1 layer so they won't stick together.
3. To make the sauce: Heat the oil in a saucepan over medium heat. Add the garlic and cook, stirring, for about 2 minutes, or until pale golden. Add the tomatoes (with juice), tomato paste, thyme, oregano, salt, and pepper. Simmer, covered, for 10 minutes.
4. To make the filling: Heat the oil in a large skillet over medium heat. Add the onion, cover, and cook, stirring often, for 3 minutes. Add the mushrooms, cover, and cook, stirring often, for 5 minutes. Add the garlic and cook, stirring, for

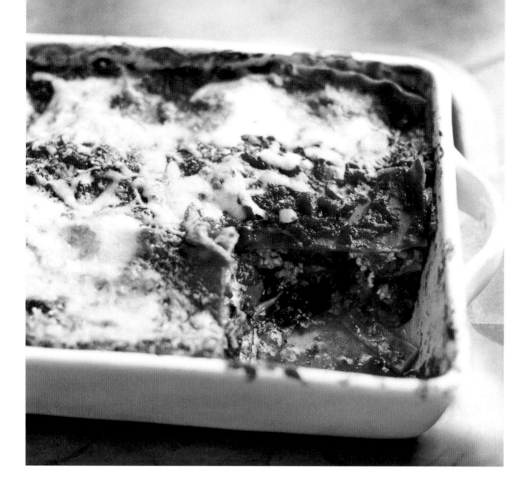

2 minutes. Add the spinach, cover, and cook for about 4 minutes, or until wilted. Season with the salt and pepper.

5. To assemble the lasagna: Spread $^1/_2$ cup of the sauce on the bottom of the prepared dish. Cover with a layer of the noodles. Spread on half of the ricotta and half of the spinach-and-mushroom filling. Spoon on one-third of the remaining sauce. Sprinkle with one-third of the mozzarella and one-third of the Parmesan. Spread half of the remaining sauce over the cheeses. Cover with a layer of noodles. Spread the remaining ricotta over the noodles. Add the remaining spinach-and-mushroom filling. Spoon half of the remaining sauce over the filling. Sprinkle with half of the remaining mozzarella and half of the remaining Parmesan. Cover with a layer of noodles. Spread the noodles with the remaining sauce.

6. Cover the dish with foil and bake for 40 minutes, or until heated through. Sprinkle the top with the remaining cheeses. Bake for 8 minutes, or until the cheeses are melted.

MUSHROOM, ONION, AND AVOCADO QUESADILLAS

PER SERVING:

381 CAL

14 g protein

36 g
carbohydrates

7 g fiber

22 g fat

6 g
saturated fat

20 mg
cholesterol

680 mg sodium

MAKES 4 SERVINGS

1 tablespoon olive oil

1 large onion, chopped

1 package (8 ounces) sliced mushrooms

¼ teaspoon salt

4 cloves garlic, minced

1 Hass avocado, mashed with a fork

2 tablespoons chopped fresh cilantro

4 flour tortillas (8" diameter)

1 cup (4 ounces) shredded reduced-fat sharp Cheddar cheese

1. Heat the oil in a large nonstick skillet over medium-high heat. Add the onion, mushrooms, and salt. Cook, stirring occasionally, for 9 to 10 minutes, or until browned. Stir in the garlic and cook for 2 minutes longer. Remove from the heat.

2. Combine the avocado and cilantro in a bowl. Arrange the tortillas in a single layer on a work surface. Spread the bottom half of each tortilla with one-fourth of the avocado mixture. Top each with 2 tablespoons of the cheese and one-fourth of the onion mixture. Sprinkle each with 2 tablespoons of the remaining cheese. Fold the top half of each tortilla over the filling.

3. Wipe out the skillet and place over medium heat. Add 2 quesadillas and cook for 3 to 4 minutes per side, or until the filling is hot and the outside is lightly browned. Repeat with the remaining quesadillas. Transfer to a cutting board and cut each in half before serving.

MACARONI AND CHEESE

MAKES 8 SERVINGS

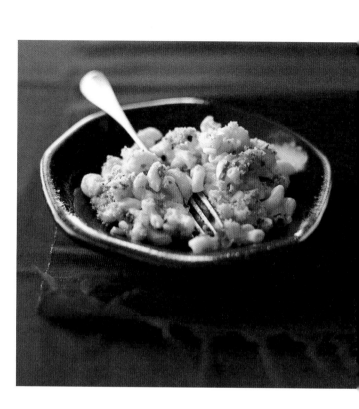

- 3 cups elbow macaroni
- 3 medium scallions, chopped (¼ cup)
- 2¼ cups 1% milk
- 3 tablespoons all-purpose flour
- 2½ cups shredded reduced-fat (2%) sharp Cheddar cheese (10 ounces)
- ½ cup reduced-fat sour cream
- 2 tablespoons Dijon mustard
- 1 teaspoon chopped chipotle chile pepper in adobo sauce
- ½ teaspoon salt
- ½ teaspoon freshly ground black pepper
- 3 tablespoons dried bread crumbs
- 2 tablespoons grated Parmesan cheese
- 2 teaspoons olive oil

1. Preheat the oven to 400°F. Coat a 2-quart baking dish with cooking spray.
2. Prepare the macaroni according to package directions.
3. Add the scallions and 1¾ cups of the milk to a large pot and bring to a simmer over medium heat while the macaroni cooks.
4. Whisk the flour and remaining ½ cup milk in a small bowl. Whisk the milk-flour mixture into the simmering milk. Cook, stirring, until thickened. Remove from the heat and gradually stir in the Cheddar until smooth. Add the sour cream, mustard, and chile pepper. Add the drained macaroni, salt, and black pepper. Transfer to the prepared baking dish.
5. Combine the bread crumbs, Parmesan, and oil in a small bowl. Sprinkle on top of the macaroni and cheese. Bake for 25 minutes, or until bubbling and golden brown.

PER SERVING:
357 CAL

19 g protein
43 g carbohydrates
2 g fiber
13 g fat
6.5 g saturated fat
35 mg cholesterol
728 mg sodium

Notes: *Be sure to wear plastic gloves when handling fresh or dried chile peppers.*

This recipe has a higher percentage of carbs than most, so consider it a special indulgence.

ROASTED RATATOUILLE WITH BEANS AND CHEESE

295 CAL

13 g protein
34 g carbohydrates
9 g fiber
13 g total fat
3 g saturated fat
344 mg sodium

MAKES 4 SERVINGS

1 onion, chopped

1 eggplant, peeled and cut into 1" pieces

1 zucchini, peeled and cut into 1" pieces

1 red bell pepper, cut into 1" pieces

2 tablespoons canola oil

1 can (15 ounces) no-salt-added chickpeas, rinsed and drained

1 cup marinara sauce

1 tablespoon balsamic vinegar

3/4 cup part-skim ricotta cheese

1. Preheat the oven to 400°F. Coat a baking sheet with cooking spray. Toss the onion, eggplant, zucchini, pepper, and oil in a large bowl. Place on the baking sheet and roast for 25 to 30 minutes, turning once, or until browned and tender.

2. Heat the chickpeas and marinara sauce in a large microwaveable bowl, covered, on high for 1 to 2 minutes, or until hot. Stir in the vinegar and roasted vegetables.

3. Divide among 4 plates and top each with 3 tablespoons of the ricotta cheese.

ASPARAGUS, RED ONION, AND TOFU STIR-FRY

MAKES 4 SERVINGS

PER SERVING:
222 CAL

13 g protein	
15 g carbohydrates	
4 g fiber	
13 g fat	
1 g saturated fat	
219 mg sodium	

- ½ cup vegetable broth
- 1 tablespoon molasses
- 1 tablespoon reduced-sodium soy sauce
- 2 teaspoons grated fresh ginger
- 2 cloves garlic, finely chopped
- 1 package (14 ounces) firm tofu, drained and cut into ½" cubes
- 2 teaspoons cornstarch
- 2 tablespoons canola oil
- 1 pound asparagus, diagonally cut into 2" pieces
- ½ red onion, thinly sliced
- 1 tablespoon ground flaxseed
- 2 teaspoons toasted sesame seeds

1. Combine the broth, molasses, soy sauce, ginger, and garlic in a 13" × 9" ceramic baking dish. Whisk. Place the tofu in a single layer in the marinade. Toss gently. Set aside to marinate for 30 minutes, tossing occasionally.

2. Remove the tofu with a slotted spoon, then whisk the cornstarch into the marinade.

3. Heat a large nonstick skillet or wok over medium-high heat. Add 1 tablespoon of the oil and heat for 1 minute. Add the asparagus and onion. Cook, tossing, for 3 to 4 minutes, or until crisp-tender. Remove to a tray. Return the pan to the heat. Add the remaining 1 tablespoon oil and heat. Place the reserved tofu in the pan. Cook, without tossing, for 1 minute, or until browned on the bottom. Toss. Cook for 2 minutes more, or until all sides are browned. Return the asparagus and onion to the pan and add the flaxseed along with the marinade. Toss for 1 minute, or until thickened. Serve sprinkled with the sesame seeds.

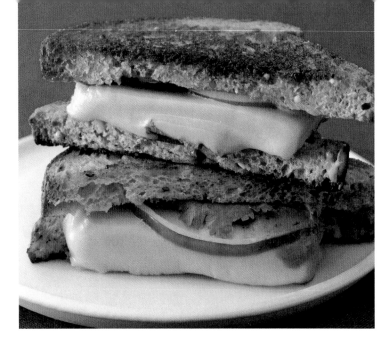

CHIPOTLE GRILLED CHEESE SANDWICH

PER SERVING:

248 CAL

15 g protein

21 g
carbohydrates

2 g fiber

11 g fat

6 g
saturated fat

32 mg
cholesterol

346 mg sodium

MAKES 4 SERVINGS

1 tablespoon light mayonnaise

1 tablespoon adobo sauce from canned chipotle chiles

8 slices light extra-fiber whole wheat bread (40–45 calories each)

4 thin slices red onion

1/4 cup cilantro

1 1/2 cups (6 ounces) reduced-fat extra-sharp Cheddar cheese, sliced

1. Stir together the mayonnaise and adobo sauce in a small bowl.

2. Place 4 slices of bread on a work surface. Spread the mayonnaise on the bread slices. Layer with the onion, cilantro, and cheese and top with the remaining bread slices.

3. Coat the top bread slice of each sandwich with cooking spray. Place the coated side down on the grill pan or skillet. Coat the remaining bread slice of each sandwich with cooking spray. Place a heavy pan over the top of the sandwiches. Cook for 2 minutes, then turn and repeat.

Note: *A panini or sandwich press works well for making these sandwiches, although an indoor grill (George Foreman) will also do the trick. Place the sandwiches (coated with cooking spray) on the press or grill, close the lid, and press slightly. There's no need to turn the sandwiches.*

VEGETARIAN CURRY BURGERS

MAKES 6 SERVINGS

PER SERVING:
169 CAL

6 g protein	
18 g carbohydrates	
5 g fiber	
9 g fat	
1 g saturated fat	
0 mg cholesterol	
18 mg sodium	

- 2 tablespoons olive or canola oil
- 1 medium onion, chopped (about 1 cup)
- 1 teaspoon curry powder
- 1/2 teaspoon ground coriander
- 1/2 teaspoon crushed fennel seeds
- 1 1/2 cups white button mushrooms, chopped
- 1 1/2 cups cooked and drained chickpeas
- 1 medium carrot, grated (about 1 cup)
- 1/4 cup chopped walnuts
- 3 tablespoons chopped cilantro
- 1/2 teaspoon salt
- 1/4 teaspoon ground black pepper

1. Warm 1 tablespoon of the oil in a medium nonstick skillet over medium-high heat. Add the onion, curry powder, coriander, and fennel. Cook, stirring frequently, for about 2 minutes, or until the onion starts to soften. Add the mushrooms and stir to mix. Cover and cook for about 4 minutes longer, or until the liquid pools in the pan. Uncover and cook for about 3 minutes more, or until the liquid is evaporated.
2. Transfer the mixture to the bowl of a food processor fitted with a metal blade. Add the chickpeas. Pulse until well chopped. Transfer to a bowl. Add the carrot, walnuts, cilantro, salt, and pepper and mix well.
3. Lightly dust hands with flour. Shape the mixture into six 4"-wide patties.
4. Warm the remaining 1 tablespoon oil in a large skillet over medium heat. Place the patties in the pan. Cook for about 4 minutes, or until browned on the bottom. Flip and cook for about 4 minutes longer, or until heated through.

CHICKEN AND TURKEY DISHES

PESTO CHICKEN BAKE

MAKES 4 SERVINGS

2$\frac{1}{2}$ pounds chicken thighs or drumsticks
1$\frac{1}{2}$ pounds baby potatoes
  1 pint cherry tomatoes
 $\frac{1}{2}$ cup pesto
  2 tablespoons water
  2 teaspoons olive oil
    Salt
    Freshly ground black pepper

1. Preheat the oven to 425°F.
2. In a large roasting pan, mix together the chicken, potatoes, tomatoes, pesto, water, and oil and salt and pepper to season. Bake for 45 minutes.

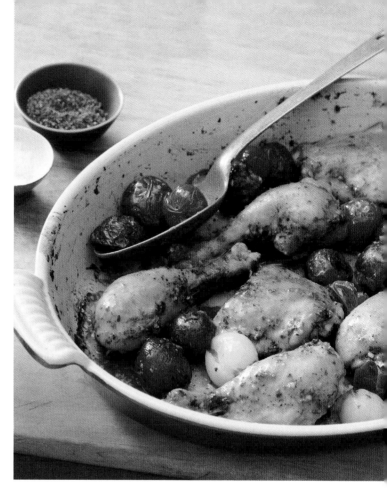

PER SERVING:
666 CAL

66 g protein

35 g
carbohydrates

4 g fiber

28 g fat

7 g
saturated fat

245 mg
cholesterol

641 mg sodium

CHICKEN WITH WHITE WINE AND PARSLEY

PER SERVING:

281 CAL

27 g protein	
8 g carbohydrates	
0.5 g fiber	
12 g fat	
2 g saturated fat	
66 mg cholesterol	
77 mg sodium	

MAKES 4 SERVINGS

¼ cup all-purpose flour

1 pound thin-sliced boneless, skinless chicken breasts

3 tablespoons olive oil

¾ cup white wine or reduced-sodium chicken broth

1 tablespoon freshly squeezed lemon juice (from ½ lemon)

Salt

Freshly ground black pepper

2 tablespoons roughly chopped flat-leaf parsley

1. Put the flour on a plate and dip the chicken into it to coat both sides.
2. Heat 1 tablespoon of the oil in a medium nonstick skillet over medium-high heat. When the oil is hot, add one-third of the chicken and cook for 2 to 3 minutes per side. Remove to plates. Repeat twice with the remaining oil and chicken.
3. Pour the wine or broth and lemon juice into the pan. Cook over high heat until about ¼ cup remains. Season with the salt and pepper to taste. Stir in the parsley and spoon the sauce around the chicken.

Note: *You can make this the Italian way, with veal scaloppine, but less-expensive chicken works perfectly. It's lightly crisped and juicy, with just enough sauce to flavor each bite.*

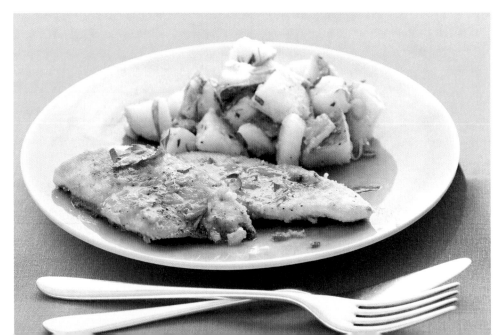

DOUBLE ROASTED CHICKEN

MAKES 4 SERVINGS

1 quartered chicken (2$\frac{1}{2}$ pounds), skin removed

$\frac{1}{2}$ cup olive oil

2 tablespoons freshly squeezed lemon juice (from 1 lemon)

$\frac{3}{4}$ teaspoon salt

$\frac{1}{4}$ teaspoon freshly ground black pepper

4 large onions, sliced

4 large pitas (6$\frac{1}{2}$" each)

2 tablespoons pine nuts, toasted

PER SERVING:

759 CAL

56 g protein	
49 g carbohydrates	
4 g fiber	
37 g fat	
5 g saturated fat	
155 mg cholesterol	
943 mg sodium	

1. Preheat the oven to 400°F.
2. Put the chicken on a rimmed baking sheet.
3. Mix the oil, lemon juice, salt, and pepper in a small bowl. Brush about $\frac{1}{4}$ cup of the mixture over the chicken.
4. Roast the chicken for about 20 minutes, or until it is nearly done.
5. While the chicken is roasting, add the onions to the remaining oil mixture and toss to coat thoroughly.
6. Heat a large skillet over medium-high heat. Add the onion mixture and cook for 8 to 10 minutes, or until the onions are golden brown.
7. Remove the chicken from the oven and arrange the pitas on the baking sheet. Scatter half of the onions onto the pitas, and place a chicken quarter on each. Roast for 10 to 15 minutes longer, or until a thermometer inserted in the thickest portion registers 165°F. Remove from the oven, top with the remaining onions, and sprinkle with the nuts. Season to taste with more salt and pepper and additional lemon juice, if desired.

CURRIED CHICKEN-AND-BROCCOLI CASSEROLE

MAKES 6 SERVINGS

- 1 pound broccoli florets
- $1/4$ cup water
- 1 can reduced-sodium cream of mushroom soup
- $1/4$ cup mayonnaise
- 1 tablespoon freshly squeezed lemon juice (from $1/2$ lemon)
- $1^{1}/_{2}$ teaspoons curry powder
- $1/2$ teaspoon salt
- $1/2$ teaspoon ground black pepper
- $1^{1}/_{2}$ pounds boneless, skinless chicken breasts, cut into bite-size chunks
- $1/4$ cup shredded reduced-fat Colby or Swiss cheese

1. Preheat the oven to 350°F. Coat a 13″ × 9″ baking dish with cooking spray. Set aside.
2. Place the broccoli and water in a large resealable plastic storage bag. Microwave on high power, rotating occasionally, for about 3 to 5 minutes, or until bright green. Drain and set aside.
3. Mix the soup, mayonnaise, lemon juice, curry powder, salt, and pepper in a small bowl. Line the baking dish with the reserved broccoli. Top with the chicken. Cover evenly with the soup mixture. Sprinkle with the cheese. Cover and bake for about 25 minutes. Uncover and bake for 15 to 20 minutes longer, or until golden and bubbling.

BUTTERMILK "FRIED" CHICKEN

MAKES 4 SERVINGS

PER SERVING:
364 CAL

47 g protein
25 g carbohydrates
1 g fiber
7.5 g fat
1.5 g saturated fat
135 mg cholesterol
951 mg sodium

- $\frac{1}{3}$ cup all-purpose flour
- 2 teaspoons fresh thyme or 1 teaspoon dried
- $\frac{3}{4}$ teaspoon salt
- $\frac{1}{4}$ teaspoon freshly ground black pepper
- $\frac{1}{2}$ cup 1% buttermilk
- 1 egg white
- $\frac{3}{4}$ cup seasoned dried bread crumbs (we used Progresso)
- 1 cut-up whole chicken (about $3\frac{1}{2}$ pounds), skin removed
- 1 lemon, cut into wedges (optional)

1. Preheat the oven to 400°F. Coat a baking sheet with oil and set aside.
2. Combine the flour, thyme, salt, and pepper in a shallow dish and mix with a fork.
3. Pour the buttermilk into another shallow dish and whisk in the egg white. Put the bread crumbs in a third shallow dish.
4. Dredge a piece of chicken in the flour and shake off the excess. Using tongs, dip the chicken into the buttermilk to coat and then transfer to the dish with the bread crumbs. Coat the chicken evenly with the crumbs and put on the prepared pan. Repeat with the remaining chicken pieces.
5. Bake the chicken for 35 to 40 minutes, or until the crumbs are golden brown and the chicken is cooked through. Garnish with the lemon wedges, if desired, and serve immediately.

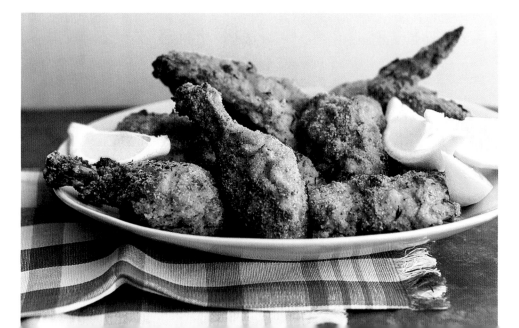

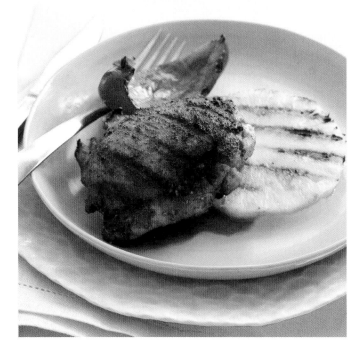

JERK CHICKEN IN A JIFFY

PER SERVING:

318 CAL

| 34 g protein |
| 10 g carbohydrates |
| 1 g fiber |
| 15 g fat |
| 2.5 g saturated fat |
| 141 mg cholesterol |
| 467 mg sodium |

MAKES 4 SERVINGS

   Red bell pepper, quartered

4 thick pineapple slices

2½ tablespoons canola oil

   Salt

1½ tablespoons jerk seasoning

4 large boneless, skinless chicken thighs (about 1½ pounds)

1. Oil the grate and heat the grill to medium-high.
2. Toss the pepper and pineapple in a medium bowl with 1 tablespoon of the oil to coat. Remove and sprinkle the pepper with the salt. In the same bowl, combine the jerk seasoning and the remaining 1½ tablespoons oil. Add the chicken and toss to coat.
3. Grill the chicken, pepper, and pineapple for about 10 minutes, turning once.

CHICKEN PERSONAL PIZZA

MAKES 1 PIZZA

- 1 whole wheat pita, toasted
- ½ cup chopped tomatoes
- ¼ cup shredded part-skim mozzarella
- ½ cup grilled chicken breast
- ¼ cup chopped sun-dried tomatoes
- 1 teaspoon minced garlic
- ¼ teaspoon oregano

1. Top the pita with the chopped tomatoes, cheese, chicken, and sun-dried tomatoes. Sprinkle with the garlic and oregano.
2. Place under the oven broiler for 5 to 8 minutes, or until bubbly.

PER SERVING:
352 CAL

39 g protein	
36 g carbohydrates	
12 g fiber	
9 g fat	
2.3 g saturated fat	
60 mg cholesterol	
720 mg sodium	

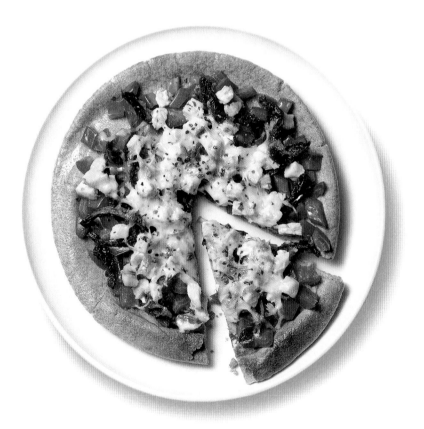

CHICKEN SOFT TACOS
WITH TANGY GUACAMOLE

PER SERVING:

421 CAL

26 g protein	
30 g carbohydrates	
7 g fiber	
23 g fat	
2.5 g saturated fat	
55 mg cholesterol	
477 mg sodium	

MAKES 6 SERVINGS

- $\frac{1}{4}$ cup + 2 tablespoons vegetable oil
- 3 cloves garlic, halved
- 2 small serrano chile peppers or 1 small jalapeño chile pepper, halved
- $\frac{1}{2}$ cup loosely packed cilantro
- $\frac{1}{3}$ cup freshly squeezed lime juice (from 2 limes)
- $\frac{1}{4}$ teaspoon freshly ground black pepper
- 1 teaspoon salt
- 4 boneless, skinless chicken breast halves (about $1\frac{1}{4}$ pounds)
- 1 large white onion, sliced $\frac{1}{4}$" thick
- 2 ripe Hass avocados
- 12 corn tortillas (6" diameter)

1. Heat $\frac{1}{4}$ cup of the oil in a small skillet over medium heat. Add the garlic and serrano chile peppers or jalapeño chile pepper and cook, stirring frequently, for 1 to 2 minutes, or until just browned. Process with the cilantro, lime juice, black pepper, and $\frac{1}{2}$ teaspoon of the salt in a blender or food processor until smooth.

2. Put the chicken in a shallow dish and spread half of the garlic mixture over all sides of the chicken.

3. Heat 1 tablespoon of the remaining oil in a large skillet over medium-high heat. Add the onion and cook, stirring occasionally, for about 5 minutes, or until golden but still slightly crunchy. Chop enough of the onion to make $\frac{1}{4}$ cup and set aside. Put the rest of the onion on a plate. Set aside the skillet.

4. Peel and pit the avocados and put the flesh in a bowl. Add the reserved chopped onion, $\frac{1}{4}$ teaspoon of the salt, and remaining garlic mixture. Coarsely mash with a potato masher or fork.

5. Return the skillet to medium heat and add the remaining 1 tablespoon oil. Lift each chicken breast half and let the excess marinade drip off. Discard the extra marinade. Add the chicken to the hot pan and sprinkle with the remaining $\frac{1}{4}$ teaspoon salt. Brown on one side, about 5 minutes, then flip and finish cooking for 3 to 4 minutes longer. Remove to a cutting board. Put the reserved sliced onion in the skillet to reheat. Scrape up any brown bits stuck to the bottom of the pan.

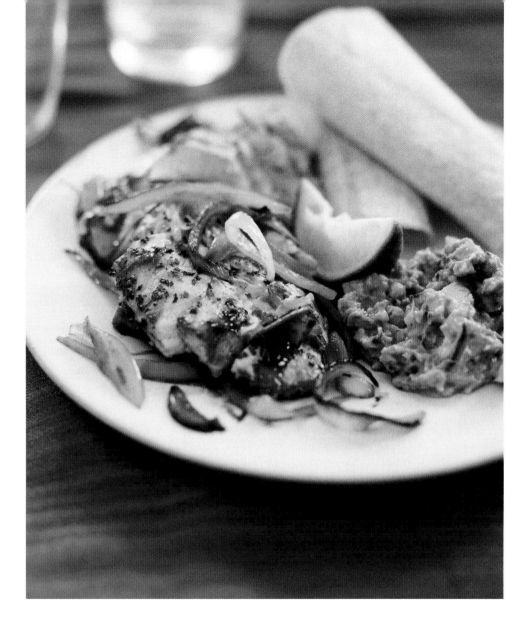

6. Wrap the tortillas in damp paper towels and microwave on high power for 1 minute. Remove the paper towels and keep the tortillas warm. Cut the chicken across the grain into $1/4"$ slices and toss with the onion in the pan. Serve with the tortillas and guacamole.

Note: *Be sure to wear plastic gloves when handling fresh or dried chile peppers.*

Tip: *You can complete all the elements of these tacos hours before serving. Press plastic wrap directly onto the guacamole so it won't brown. Slice the chicken and put it in the skillet with the onions, ready to reheat.*

ROTINI WITH TURKEY SAUSAGE AND BROCCOLI

MAKES 4 SERVINGS

- 2 cooked Italian-style turkey sausages, sliced
- 1 ripe tomato, diced
- 2 cups cooked broccoli
- ½ cup shredded part-skim mozzarella
- 1½ tablespoons olive oil
- ¾ teaspoon dried thyme
- ¼ teaspoon salt
- ¼ teaspoon freshly ground black pepper
- 3 cups hot cooked rotini

1. Stir together the sausages, tomato, broccoli, cheese, oil, thyme, salt and pepper in a medium bowl.
2. Mix in the rotini.

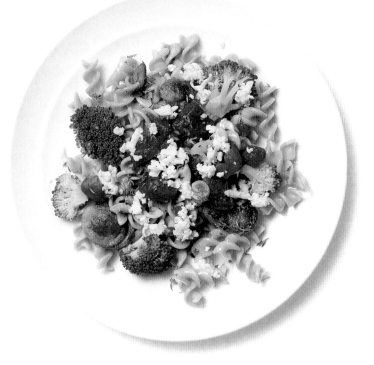

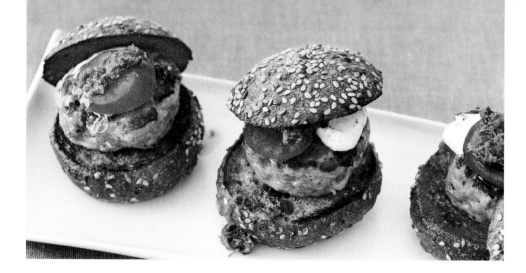

PIZZA-STYLE TURKEY SLIDERS

MAKES 4 SERVINGS (2 SLIDERS EACH)

1 slice whole wheat bread, torn into pieces

2 large egg whites

1/4 cup pesto sauce

12 ounces extra-lean (97–99% fat free) ground turkey breast

1/2 medium carrot, grated (1/4 cup)

1/8 medium sweet onion, finely chopped (1/4 cup)

1/4 teaspoon freshly ground black pepper

1/8 teaspoon salt

2 ounces fresh mozzarella, cut into 8 slices

8 whole grain rolls (1.3 ounces each), split and toasted

2 plum tomatoes, cut into 4 slices each

1. Preheat the broiler. Coat the broiler pan rack with cooking spray and line the broiler pan with foil.

2. Mix the bread, egg whites, and 3 tablespoons of the pesto in a medium bowl. Let stand for 5 minutes, or until the bread is softened. Mash with a fork.

3. Add the turkey, carrot, onion, pepper, and salt. Mix well but with a light hand. Form into 8 patties, using a slightly heaping 1/4 cup for each.

4. Place the patties on the prepared broiler pan. Broil 2" to 4" from the heat, turning once, for about 10 minutes, or until browned and no longer pink in the thickest part. Top each with a slice of the cheese and broil for 1 minute longer to melt.

5. Put the bun bottoms on a serving plate. Top each with a burger and a tomato slice. Dab evenly with the remaining 1 tablespoon pesto. Top with the other halves of the buns.

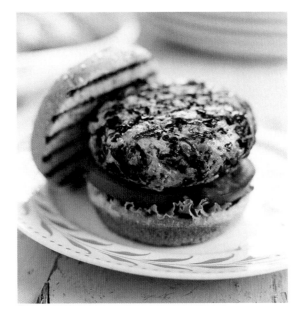

TURKEY-SPINACH BURGERS

PER SERVING:

305 CAL

29 g protein	
30 g carbohydrates	
6 g fiber	
9.5 g fat	
2.5 g saturated fat	
65 mg cholesterol	
723 mg sodium	

MAKES 4 SERVINGS

- 1 pound ground lean turkey breast (7% fat or leaner)
- 1 package (10 ounces) frozen chopped spinach, thawed and water squeezed out
- 2 tablespoons barbecue sauce
- 1/2 teaspoon salt
- 1/4 teaspoon freshly ground black pepper
- 4 whole wheat hamburger buns, toasted
- 4 tomato slices
- 4 lettuce leaves

1. Heat the grill to medium-high and coat the rack with cooking spray.
2. Combine the turkey, spinach, barbecue sauce, salt, and pepper in a large bowl. Shape the mixture into four 3 1/2"-diameter patties.
3. Grill the patties for 10 to 12 minutes, turning once, or until a meat thermometer inserted into the middle from the side registers 165°F. Serve on the buns with the tomato and lettuce.

Note: *For a Tex-Mex burger, substitute 2 tablespoons canned chopped green chile peppers, drained, for the barbecue sauce and add 1 teaspoon chili powder.*

ORANGE-SESAME TURKEY CUTLETS

MAKES 4 SERVINGS

- 1 cup orange juice
- 1 tablespoon reduced-sodium soy sauce
- 1 teaspoon dark sesame oil
- 1 teaspoon minced garlic
- 1 pound turkey cutlets
- 1 teaspoon cornstarch
- ¾ cup reduced-sodium chicken broth
- 1 tablespoon minced fresh cilantro

PER SERVING:

165 CAL

29 g protein	
8 g carbohydrates	
0 g fiber	
2 g fat	
0 g saturated fat	
45 mg cholesterol	
329 mg sodium	

1. Combine the orange juice, soy sauce, oil, and garlic in a zip-top bag. Add the turkey and chill for 1 hour.
2. Coat a nonstick skillet with cooking spray and heat over medium-high heat. Add the turkey (reserving the marinade). Cook, turning once, for about 4 minutes, or until browned. Remove to a plate.
3. Mix the cornstarch and broth in a bowl. Stir in the reserved marinade. Reduce the heat to medium and add to the skillet. Cook, stirring, for 3 minutes, or until thickened. Add the turkey and cook for about 5 minutes, or until done. Top with the cilantro.

To freeze: *Pack the cooled cooked cutlets and sauce in a freezer-quality plastic container. To use, thaw overnight in the refrigerator. Cover and microwave on high power for 5 minutes, or until hot.*

BEEF, PORK, AND LAMB DISHES

BRONZED LONDON BROIL

MAKES 6 SERVINGS

- 1 tablespoon olive oil
- 1 medium onion, chopped
- 3 cloves garlic, minced
- 1 teaspoon red-pepper flakes
- 1 teaspoon ground cinnamon
- $2/3$ cup diced canned tomatoes
- $1/2$ cup brewed coffee
- $1/4$ cup Worcestershire sauce
- 2 tablespoons balsamic vinegar
- $1/4$ cup light molasses
- Salt
- Freshly ground black pepper
- 1 London broil (about 2 pounds, 1" thick)

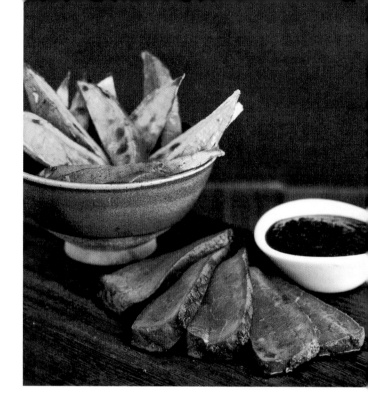

1. Heat the oil in a large nonstick skillet over medium-high heat. Sauté the onion and garlic for about 2 minutes, or until softened. Add the pepper flakes and cinnamon and heat for 1 minute longer. Remove from the heat.
2. In a food processor, blend the onion mixture with the tomatoes, coffee, Worcestershire, vinegar, and molasses until almost smooth.
3. Return the mixture to the skillet and season with the salt and pepper. Bring to a simmer. Cook, uncovered, for 15 to 20 minutes, stirring occasionally.
4. Meanwhile, preheat the broiler, coat the broiler pan with cooking spray, and place the London broil on the pan. Brush 1 side with the sauce and broil for 7 to 9 minutes. Turn the meat over, brush with the sauce, and broil for another 7 to 9 minutes for medium-rare (an internal temperature of 145°F), or longer to desired doneness.
5. Bring the remaining sauce in the skillet to a boil for 1 minute. Slice the meat thinly and serve with the sauce on the side.

PER SERVING:
300 CAL

33 g protein
18 g carbohydrates
11 g fat
3.5 g saturated fat
50 mg cholesterol
1 g fiber
290 mg sodium

PER SERVING:

218 CAL

23 g protein	
19 g carbohydrates	
4 g fiber	
6 g fat	
2 g saturated fat	
44 mg cholesterol	
669 mg sodium	

MAKES 8 SERVINGS

MEAT LOAF

  1 ounce dried mushrooms, such as porcini

1½ cups hot water

 ½ cup bulgur

  1 can (8 ounces) tomato sauce

 ½ cup dry white wine or reduced-sodium beef broth

1½ pounds lean ground sirloin (95% lean)

  2 large egg whites, beaten lightly

  2 medium onions, finely chopped (2 cups)

  1 cup soft whole wheat bread crumbs

  2 cloves garlic, minced (1 tablespoon)

  1 teaspoon dried thyme

  1 teaspoon dried oregano

 ¾ teaspoon salt

 ½ teaspoon freshly ground black pepper

GRAVY

  2 teaspoons olive oil

  1 small onion, chopped (½ cup)

 ½ pound white mushrooms, sliced

  2 cloves garlic, minced

1½ cups reduced-sodium beef broth

 ½ cup dry white wine or ½ cup reduced-sodium beef broth

  1 teaspoon dried thyme

 ¼ teaspoon salt

  2 tablespoons water

  1 tablespoon cornstarch or arrowroot

1. To make the meat loaf: Soak the mushrooms in 1 cup of the water for 20 minutes. Drain, reserving ¼ cup of the liquid, and chop. Soak the bulgur in the remaining ½ cup water for 30 minutes, or until the liquid is absorbed.

2. Preheat the oven to 375°F. Coat a 9" × 5" × 3" loaf pan with cooking spray.

3. Combine the mushrooms, reserved mushroom liquid, and bulgur in a large bowl. Add the tomato sauce, reserving 1 tablespoon for the gravy, along with

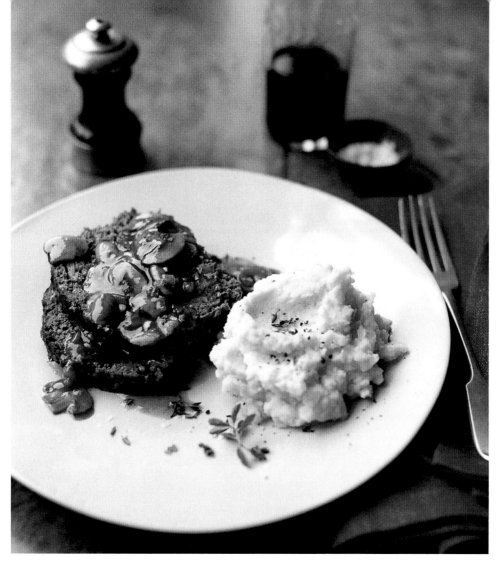

the wine or broth, sirloin, egg whites, onions, bread crumbs, garlic, thyme, oregano, salt, and pepper. Gently mix to combine. Transfer the mixture to the prepared pan. Bake for 1 hour 15 minutes.

4. To make the gravy: Heat the oil in a medium skillet. Add the onion. Cook over medium heat, stirring, for 3 minutes. Add the mushrooms and stir for 5 minutes. Add the garlic and reserved tomato sauce. Cook for 1 minute. Add the broth, wine, thyme, and salt. Bring to a boil. Simmer, covered, for 10 minutes.

5. Whisk the water and cornstarch in a small bowl. Add to the gravy. Stir until thickened.

Note: *For easier slicing, let the meat loaf cool for 10 minutes before serving.*

SPICY CHIPOTLE BEEF

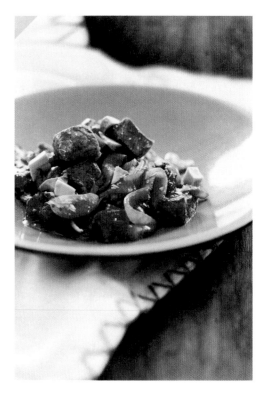

PER SERVING:
345 CAL

30 g protein	
18 g carbohydrates	
4 g fiber	
15 g fat	
3 g saturated fat	
75 mg cholesterol	
839 mg sodium	

MAKES 4 SERVINGS

- 2 tablespoons vegetable or olive oil
- 1 pound beef tenderloin, strip, or sirloin, cut into 1" cubes
- 1 large white onion, sliced ½" thick
- 4 cloves garlic, minced
- ½ cup dark beer, broth, or water
- 2 tablespoons Worcestershire sauce
- 2 cans (14.5 ounces each) no-salt-added diced tomatoes, drained
- 12 ounces shiitake, oyster, or other mushrooms or a combination, stemmed and sliced ¼" thick
- 2 canned chipotle chile peppers in adobo sauce, chopped
- 1 teaspoon salt
- ⅓ cup chopped cilantro

1. Heat the oil in a Dutch oven over high heat. When hot, add the beef in an uncrowded single layer. Cook, stirring frequently to brown all sides, for about 4 minutes for medium-rare, or until almost at desired doneness. Remove to the plate, leaving the oil behind.
2. Return the pan to medium-high heat. Add the onion. Cook, stirring occasionally, for about 7 minutes, or until browned. Add the garlic and stir for 1 minute. Add the beer, broth, or water and Worcestershire. Add the tomatoes, mushrooms, peppers, and salt and cook, stirring occasionally and scraping up the bits stuck to the bottom of the pan, for about 10 minutes, or until the mushrooms are done and the liquid is reduced to a sauce.
3. Season with more salt, if desired. Return the meat to the pan and heat. Serve sprinkled with the cilantro.

Get ahead: *You can prepare this early on the day you plan to serve it. Refrigerate the sauce and meat separately, then bring them back to room temperature before reheating. Warm the sauce first and add the meat just long enough to heat through.*

BEEF-AND-POTATO PIE

MAKES 4 SERVINGS

- 1 pound lean ground beef
- 1 teaspoon oil
- 1 teaspoon ground chipotle chile pepper or 1 tablespoon chili powder
- ³⁄₄ teaspoon salt
  Freshly ground black pepper
- 1 can (14.75 ounces) cream-style corn
- 1 can (11 ounces) Mexican-style whole kernel corn, drained
- 2¹⁄₂ cups mashed potatoes

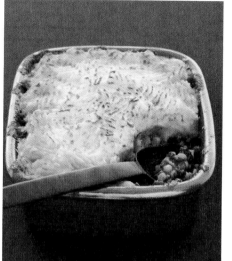

PER SERVING:

455 CAL

| 36 g protein |
| 46 g carbohydrates |
| 4 g fiber |
| 15 g fat |
| 5 g saturated fat |
| 91 mg cholesterol |
| 901 mg sodium |

1. Preheat the oven to 375°F.
2. Brown the beef in the oil. Season with the chile pepper or chili powder, salt, and black pepper to taste. Add the cream-style corn and whole kernel corn. Pour into a baking dish. Spread the potatoes over the top. Bake for 15 to 20 minutes, or until bubbly around the edges, and then broil for 2 to 3 minutes to brown the top.

Note: *Be sure to wear plastic gloves when handling fresh or dried chile peppers.*

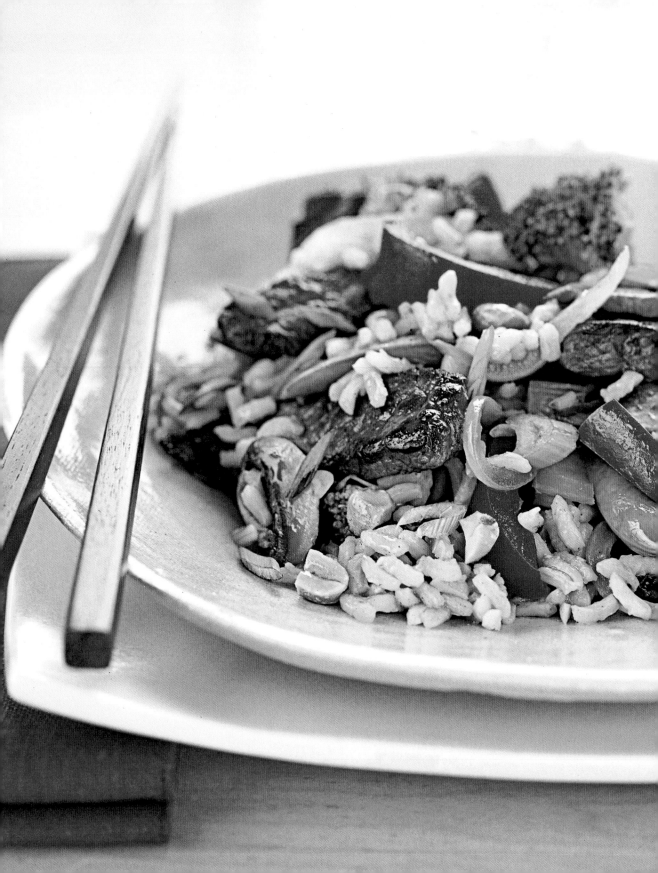

STIR-FRIED RICE
WITH ASIAN VEGETABLES AND BEEF

MAKES 4 SERVINGS

- 8 ounces sirloin or top round steak, $3/4$" thick, thinly sliced
- 2 tablespoons reduced-sodium soy sauce
- 2 teaspoons canola or other vegetable oil
- 1 bag (14 ounces) frozen stir-fry or Asian vegetable mix
- 1 pouch (10 ounces) frozen brown rice
- 1 tablespoon finely chopped fresh ginger
- 2 teaspoons finely minced garlic
- $1/2$ cup diagonally sliced scallions
- $1/4$ cup coarsely chopped dry-roasted peanuts

PER SERVING:

270 CAL

18 g protein

23 g
carbohydrates

11 g fat

2.5 g
saturated fat

35 mg
cholesterol

4 g fiber

530 mg sodium

1. Toss the steak with 1 tablespoon of the soy sauce.
2. Heat a wok or large skillet over high heat. Add the oil. Place the steak in a single layer and cook without stirring for about 1 minute, or until browned. Cook another minute, stirring once or twice, until all of the pink is gone. With a slotted spoon or tongs, transfer the meat to a dish and set aside.
3. Add the vegetables to the skillet's juices and stir-fry over medium heat for about 5 minutes, or until the vegetables are tender.
4. Cook the rice according to the package directions.
5. Add the ginger and garlic to the skillet and stir-fry for 30 seconds. Add the steak, cooked rice, scallions, peanuts, and remaining 1 tablespoon soy sauce. Stir-fry until heated through.

Note: *Slice the meat when partially frozen. It's quicker and easier than cutting it when it has thawed.*

STEAK QUESADILLAS

PER SERVING:

405 CAL

26 g protein	
39 g carbohydrates	
8 g fiber	
21 g fat	
8 g saturated fat	
58 mg cholesterol	
1,011 mg sodium	

MAKES 4 SERVINGS

- 1 small red onion
- ½ avocado
- 1 teaspoon olive oil
- 8 ounces strip steak
- 4 100-calorie tortillas
- 1 cup salsa
- 1 cup canned black beans, rinsed and drained
- 1 cup Monterey Jack cheese

1. Slice the onion and avocado.
2. Heat the oil in a skillet. Cook the steak and divide among the tortillas. Top with the avocado, onion, and ¼ cup each salsa, black beans, and cheese. Heat in the skillet.

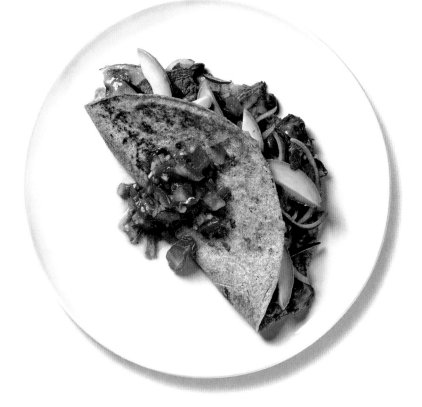

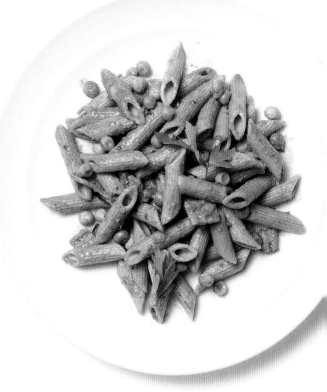

PENNE À LA VODKA

MAKES 4 SERVINGS

- 2 tablespoons butter
- 4 slices Canadian bacon, diced
- 2 tablespoons tomato paste
- 1 tablespoon parsley
- 4 tablespoons cream
- ¼ cup vodka
- 3 cups cooked penne

1. Melt the butter in a skillet. Add the bacon, tomato paste, and parsley. Cook for 10 minutes. Add the cream and vodka and cook until the vodka evaporates.
2. Toss with the penne in a serving bowl.

PER SERVING:

337 CAL

12 g protein
33 g carbohydrates
2 g fiber
14 g fat
8 g saturated fat
49 mg cholesterol
405 mg sodium

SPICY RUBBED PORK TENDERLOIN WITH EDAMAME SUCCOTASH

PER SERVING:

345 CAL

36 g protein	
30 g carbohydrates	
7 g fiber	
9 g fat	
3 g saturated fat	
80 mg cholesterol	
108 mg sodium	

MAKES 4 SERVINGS

- $1/2$ teaspoon chili powder
- $1/2$ teaspoon ground cumin
- $1/4$ teaspoon smoked paprika
- $1/4$ teaspoon garlic powder
- 1 pork tenderloin (about 1 pound)
- 2 cups frozen or fresh shelled edamame
- $1/3$ cup light sour cream
- 2 tablespoons freshly squeezed lime juice (from 1 lime)
- 2 cups frozen corn kernels, thawed
- 1 medium tomato, seeded and chopped
- $1/4$ cup chopped fresh cilantro

1. Preheat the oven to 425°F. Combine the chili powder, cumin, paprika, and garlic powder in a small bowl.
2. Place the pork in a roasting pan and coat with the spice mixture. Roast, turning once, for 25 minutes, or until a thermometer inserted in the center reaches 155°F. Let stand for 10 minutes. Cut diagonally into 12 slices.
3. Meanwhile, cook the edamame according to the package directions. Rinse under cold running water and drain.
4. Stir together the sour cream and lime juice in a medium bowl. Add the edamame, corn, tomato, and cilantro and stir. Divide the salad among 4 shallow bowls. Serve with the pork slices.

BBQ PORK CHOPS

MAKES 4 SERVINGS

- 2 tablespoons ketchup
- 1 tablespoon Dijon mustard
- 2 teaspoons honey
- 1 teaspoon olive oil
- 1 teaspoon reduced-sodium soy sauce
- $\frac{1}{2}$ teaspoon balsamic vinegar
- $\frac{1}{2}$ teaspoon salt
- $\frac{1}{4}$ teaspoon freshly ground black pepper
- 4 bone-in, $\frac{3}{4}$"-thick pork rib chops

PER SERVING:
204 CAL

30 g protein
6 g carbohydrates
0 g fiber
6 g fat
2 g saturated fat
92 mg cholesterol
577 mg sodium

1. Combine the ketchup, mustard, honey, oil, soy sauce, vinegar, salt, and pepper in a small bowl and beat with a fork to make the barbecue sauce.
2. Heat a large nonstick skillet over high heat. Spray the pan with oil and brown the pork chops for about 2 minutes on each side. Reduce the heat to medium.
3. Coat the tops and sides of the pork chops with half of the sauce. Turn and coat the other side with the remaining sauce.
4. Cook for about 3 minutes, turning once.

Save time: *Use the same teaspoon for the honey that you used for the oil. The honey will slide right off the slick spoon, and you'll have just one utensil to wash.*

PORK STIR-FRY WITH GARLIC BROCCOLI

PER SERVING:

240 CAL

28 g protein

12 g
carbohydrates

4 g fiber

9 g fat

3 g
saturated fat

75 mg
cholesterol

290 mg sodium

MAKES 4 SERVINGS

3 cups broccoli, cut into 1" pieces

1/2 cup chopped scallions

2 tablespoons chopped garlic

2 tablespoons peeled chopped fresh ginger

3/4 cup fat-free, reduced-sodium chicken broth

2 teaspoons olive oil

1 cup chopped yellow onion

1 red bell pepper, halved, seeded, and diced

1 pound boneless pork tenderloin, cut into 1/2" × 2" strips

1 tablespoon reduced-sodium soy sauce

1 tablespoon sesame seeds

1. Steam the broccoli for about 2 minutes, or until it is bright green but still firm. Rinse with cold water to stop the cooking. Drain and set aside.

2. Pulse the scallions, garlic, ginger, and 1/4 cup of the broth in a food processor until minced. Set aside.

3. Heat 1 teaspoon of the oil in a large nonstick skillet over medium-high heat. Add the onion and pepper. Sauté for 5 minutes, or until just tender. Transfer to a bowl and cover with a towel to retain the heat.

4. Add the remaining 1 teaspoon oil to the pan over medium-high heat. Add the scallion mixture and sauté for about 1 minute, stirring. Add the pork and soy sauce and sauté for 4 minutes, or until the pork is nearly cooked.

5. Add the remaining 1/2 cup broth and bring to a boil. Add the reserved broccoli to the skillet and stir for about 3 minutes, or until the broccoli is cooked through. Add the onion and pepper back to the pan. Garnish with the sesame seeds.

FAST LAMB CURRY

MAKES 4 SERVINGS

- 1 pound ground lamb
- 5 teaspoons curry powder
- 1/2 teaspoon salt
- 1/2 cup water
- 15 ounces fresh marinara sauce
- 6 ounces baby spinach
- Freshly ground black pepper

Brown the lamb with the curry powder and salt in a large skillet. Stir in the water, marinara sauce, and spinach. Simmer, uncovered, for 5 minutes. Season with more salt and the pepper to taste.

Note: *Serve with naan (Indian flatbread) or rice, if desired.*

PER SERVING:

238 CAL

26 g protein
15 g carbohydrates
5 g fiber
8 g fat
3 g saturated fat
74 mg cholesterol
873 mg sodium

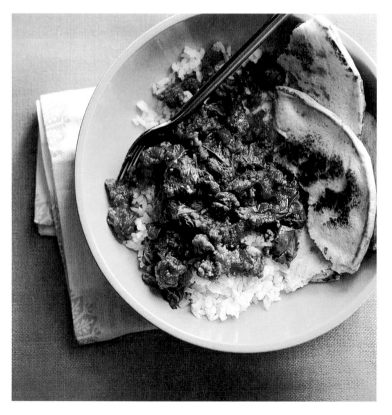

BRAISED LAMB SHANKS
WITH TOMATO-JALAPEÑO SAUCE

PER SERVING:

528 CAL

68 g protein

25 g
carbohydrates

3 g fiber

15 g fat

4 g
saturated fat

211 mg
cholesterol

904 mg sodium

MAKES 6 SERVINGS

2 tablespoons olive or vegetable oil

4 pounds lamb shanks

1 large white onion, chopped

2 jalapeño chile peppers, finely chopped

2 cans (14.5 ounces each) no-salt-added diced tomatoes

3 cups reduced-sodium beef broth

1 unpeeled head garlic, halved crosswise

1/2 teaspoon dried thyme

1/4 teaspoon salt

1 1/2 pound small red potatoes, halved

Freshly ground black pepper

1. Preheat the oven to 325°F.
2. Put the oil in a Dutch oven over medium-high heat. Sprinkle the lamb with salt, if desired. When the oil is hot, put the lamb in the pan. Cook for about 8 minutes total, or until the lamb is browned on all sides. Remove to a plate.
3. Add the onion and cook, stirring occasionally, for about 7 minutes, or until golden. Stir in the chile peppers and cook for 1 minute longer. Add the tomatoes (with juice), broth, garlic, thyme, and salt. Bring to a boil.
4. Return the lamb (and any juices) to the pan, nestling it into the liquid. Cover and bake for 1 1/2 hours. Add the potatoes and continue cooking for about 1 hour longer, or until the lamb is fork-tender and the potatoes are done.
5. Remove the lamb to a deep ovenproof serving platter. Remove and discard the garlic from the braising liquid. Using a slotted spoon, remove the potatoes from the liquid and arrange around the lamb. Cover with foil and set in the turned-off oven. Skim any excess fat from the top of the sauce. Boil the sauce over high heat to about 3 cups, or until reduced by half. Taste and season with additional salt and the black pepper, if desired. Ladle the sauce over the lamb and potatoes and serve.

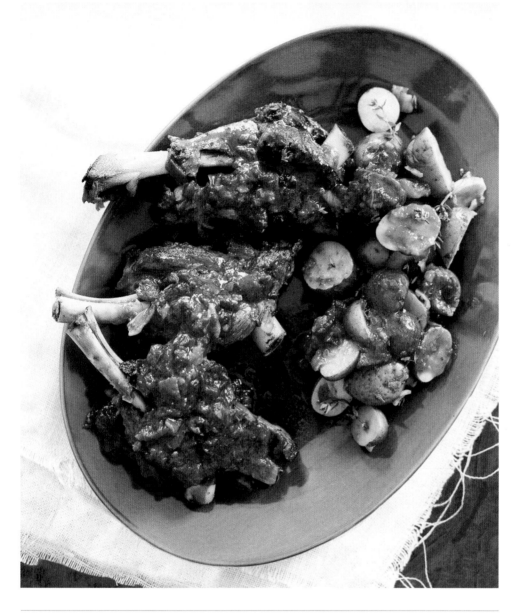

Notes: *Be sure to wear plastic gloves when handling fresh or dried chile peppers.*

Long, gentle cooking is the secret here. Check the shanks every half hour or so, and if they're boiling, reduce the temperature.

Get ahead: *Finish cooking and then refrigerate overnight right in the pot. Any excess fat can be skimmed off easily before reheating.*

FISH AND SEAFOOD DISHES

PESTO-SHRIMP TOSS

MAKES 4 SERVINGS

2	cups water
3/4	teaspoon salt
1	cup quick-cooking barley
1	package (10 ounces) broccoli florets
1 1/4	pounds raw shrimp
1–2	teaspoons vinegar
1/2	cup sun-dried tomato pesto
	Salt
	Freshly ground black pepper

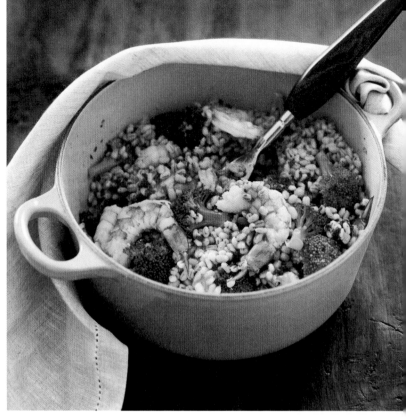

1. Bring the water and salt to a boil in a Dutch oven.
2. Stir in the barley, cover, and cook over medium heat for 5 minutes. Place the broccoli on top of the barley, cover, and cook for 5 minutes. Stir in the shrimp and vinegar, cover, and cook for 2 minutes.
3. Remove from the heat and let stand, covered, for about 4 minutes, or until the shrimp are done. Stir in the pesto and the salt and pepper to taste.

PER SERVING:
332 CAL

36 g protein
36 g carbohydrates
6 g fiber
5 g fat
1 g saturated fat
215 mg cholesterol
953 mg sodium

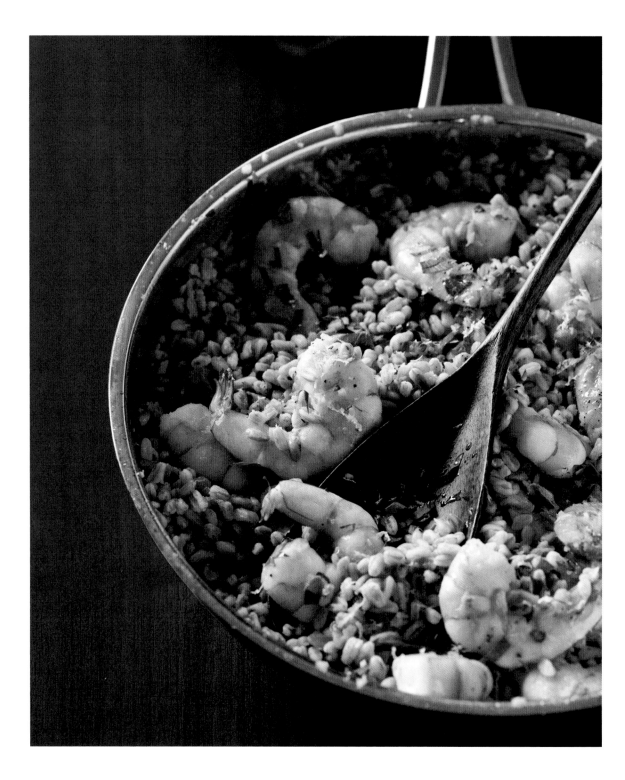

FARRO WITH SHRIMP, GARLIC, LEMON ZEST, AND PARSLEY

MAKES 4 SERVINGS

- 1 cup farro (2½ cups cooked)
- 1¾ cups water
- ½ teaspoon salt
- 2 tablespoons olive oil
- 1 pound large shrimp, shelled and deveined
- 3 cloves garlic, minced
- ¼ teaspoon freshly ground black pepper
- ¼ cup white wine or reduced-sodium chicken broth
- 3 tablespoons minced parsley
- Freshly grated zest of 2 lemons

PER SERVING:
323 CAL
25 g protein

35 g
carbohydrates

3 g fiber

8 g fat

1 g
saturated fat

168 mg
cholesterol

520 mg sodium

1. Toast the farro in a medium saucepan over medium heat for about 2 minutes, or until fragrant. Add the water and ¼ teaspoon of the salt and bring to a boil. Reduce the heat, cover, and simmer for 20 minutes. Remove from the heat and let stand for 10 minutes.

2. Heat the oil over medium-high heat in a large skillet and add the shrimp. Sauté for 1½ minutes and add the garlic, ⅛ teaspoon of the pepper, and ⅛ teaspoon of the remaining salt. Sauté for 1½ minutes longer. Pour into a bowl.

3. Add the wine or broth to the pan and scrape up anything stuck to the pan bottom. Add the farro and remaining ⅛ teaspoon salt and ⅛ teaspoon pepper and sauté, stirring frequently, for 2 minutes. Stir in the shrimp mixture, parsley, and lemon zest.

ORANGE-COCONUT SHRIMP

PER SERVING:

329 CAL

21 g protein	
23 g carbohydrates	
1 g fiber	
16 g fat	
8 g saturated fat	
151 mg cholesterol	
395 mg sodium	

MAKES 4 SERVINGS

DIP

- $1/2$ cup low-sugar or artificially sweetened orange marmalade
- 2 tablespoons spicy brown mustard
- 1 tablespoon freshly squeezed lime juice (from $1/2$ lime)

SHRIMP

- $1/2$ cup rice wine vinegar
- 2 tablespoons olive oil
- 2 teaspoons minced garlic
- $1/4$ teaspoon red-pepper flakes
- $1/4$ teaspoon salt
- $1/8$ teaspoon ground black pepper
- 1 pound jumbo shrimp, peeled, deveined, and rinsed
- $1/2$ cup unsweetened flaked coconut
- $1/4$ cup low-sugar or artificially sweetened orange marmalade

1. Preheat the oven to 350°F.
2. To make the dip: Combine the marmalade, mustard, and lime juice in a saucepan. Cook, stirring constantly, over medium heat for about 4 minutes, or until the mixture bubbles. Remove from the heat. Let stand to cool.
3. To make the shrimp: Combine the vinegar, oil, garlic, pepper flakes, salt, and black pepper in a mixing bowl. Whisk to mix. Add the shrimp. Toss to coat. Let stand for 15 minutes to marinate.
4. Meanwhile, scatter the coconut in a thin layer over a baking sheet. Bake, stirring occasionally, for about 7 minutes, or until lightly browned. Remove and let stand to cool.
5. Coat a stove-top griddle or baking sheet with cooking spray. Preheat the pan or broiler.
6. Drain the shrimp and discard the marinade. Thread 4 or 5 shrimp on each of 4 metal or soaked bamboo skewers. Cook for about 3 minutes per side, or until no longer opaque. Remove the shrimp to a tray. Brush both sides of the shrimp with the marmalade. Sprinkle with the coconut, pressing lightly to adhere. Serve with the dip.

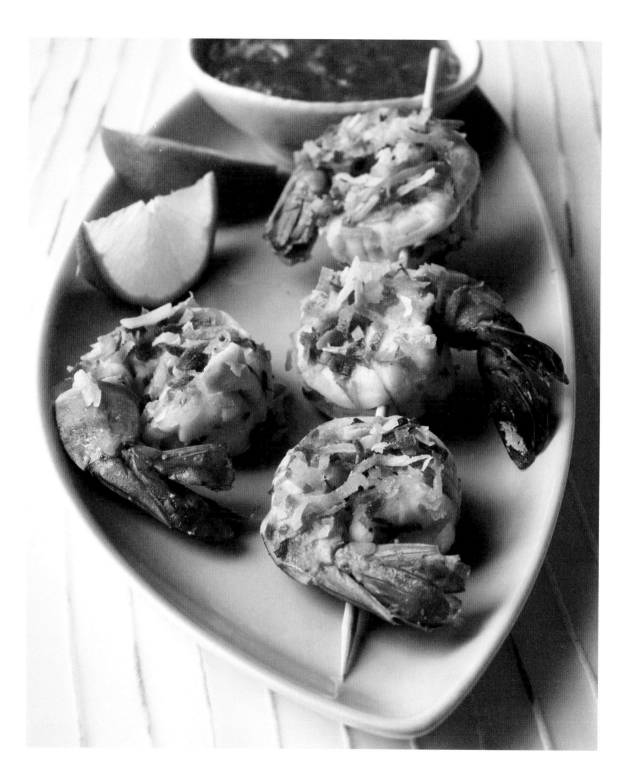

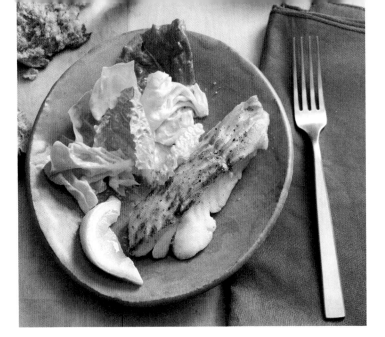

SEARED AND STEAMED FISH

PER SERVING:

160 CAL

30 g protein	
0 g carbohydrates	
0 g fiber	
3.5 g fat	
0.5 g saturated fat	
73 mg cholesterol	
92 mg sodium	

MAKES 4 SERVINGS

2 teaspoons canola oil

4 cod or other fish steaks or fillets, about 1" thick (about 6 ounces each)

Salt

Freshly ground black pepper

1. Heat the oil in a large nonstick or cast-iron skillet over medium-high heat for about 3 minutes, or until very hot. Season the fish with salt and pepper. Put in the pan and cook for about 2 minutes, or until golden brown.

2. Turn the fish and cover the pan with a tight-fitting lid. Remove the pan from the heat and let the fish steam for about 10 minutes, or until just done.

Notes: *Browned and juicy fish doesn't need fancy sauces or sides—perhaps a squirt of lemon juice and, to round out a quick dinner, a green salad and crusty bread. Flavor the fish with herbs, if you like, by topping each piece with a couple of thyme sprigs or one rosemary sprig. The steaming intensifies the herb flavor, so the fish is imbued with it. You can do the same thing with lemon slices, or top with an instant sauce. Try a spoonful of tapenade or salsa.*

You can use this technique for any medium-firm- to firm-textured fish, either steaks or fillets. We experimented with tilapia, hake, perch, sea bass, cod, halibut, salmon, swordfish, and sturgeon with excellent results.

CHILE-BAKED FISH WITH SWEET POTATOES

MAKES 4 SERVINGS

2	medium sweet potatoes (1 pound total), peeled and sliced ¼" thick
1	tablespoon vegetable oil
1¼	teaspoons salt
1	can (14.5 ounces) no-salt-added diced tomatoes
1	large clove garlic, halved
1	canned chipotle chile pepper in adobo sauce, seeded (if desired) + 1 teaspoon adobo sauce
1	teaspoon sugar
4	skinless fish fillets (about ¼ pound total), such as mahi mahi, ¾"–1" thick
2	tablespoons chopped cilantro (optional)

PER SERVING:
252 CAL

28 g protein

22 g carbohydrates

3 g fiber

5 g fat

0.5 g saturated fat

103 mg cholesterol

969 mg sodium

1. Preheat the oven to 400°F.
2. Put the potatoes in a microwaveable 8" × 8" baking dish. Drizzle with the oil and sprinkle with ½ teaspoon of the salt. Toss to coat, and spread in an even layer. Cover with plastic wrap and poke a few holes in it. Microwave on high power for 6 to 8 minutes, or until nearly tender.
3. Combine the tomatoes (with juice), garlic, pepper and sauce, sugar, and the remaining ¾ teaspoon salt in a food processor. Process to a puree, leaving a little texture.
4. Lay the fish in a single layer over the potatoes. Pour the tomato mixture evenly over the top. Bake for 15 to 20 minutes, or until the fish flakes when pressed firmly. Serve sprinkled with the cilantro, if desired.

Get ahead: *Put this quick dish together hours in advance if you'd like. Remove from the refrigerator about half an hour before baking.*

ASIAN-INSPIRED BAKED COD

PER SERVING:

310 CAL

42 g protein

12 g
carbohydrates

10 g fat

1.5 g
saturated fat

100 mg
cholesterol

2 g fiber

480 mg sodium

MAKES 4 SERVINGS

1 piece (2") fresh ginger, peeled and cut into matchsticks

1 bunch scallions, trimmed and cut into matchsticks

1 medium carrot, cut into matchsticks

3 cloves garlic, minced

4 cod fillets (about 2 pounds)

2 tablespoons chopped cilantro

1½ tablespoons reduced-sodium soy sauce

2 tablespoons ginger preserves

¼ cup water

2 tablespoons sesame oil

Cilantro sprigs

1. Preheat the oven to 400°F. Coat a 13" × 9" baking dish with cooking spray.
2. Combine the ginger, scallions, carrot, and garlic in a medium bowl and place in the prepared baking dish.
3. Place the fish over the ginger-scallion mixture. Top the fish with the cilantro.
4. Combine the soy sauce, preserves, water, and oil in a small bowl. Pour the mixture over the fish.
5. Cover and seal the dish with foil. Bake for 20 minutes, or until the fish flakes. Garnish with cilantro sprigs, if desired.

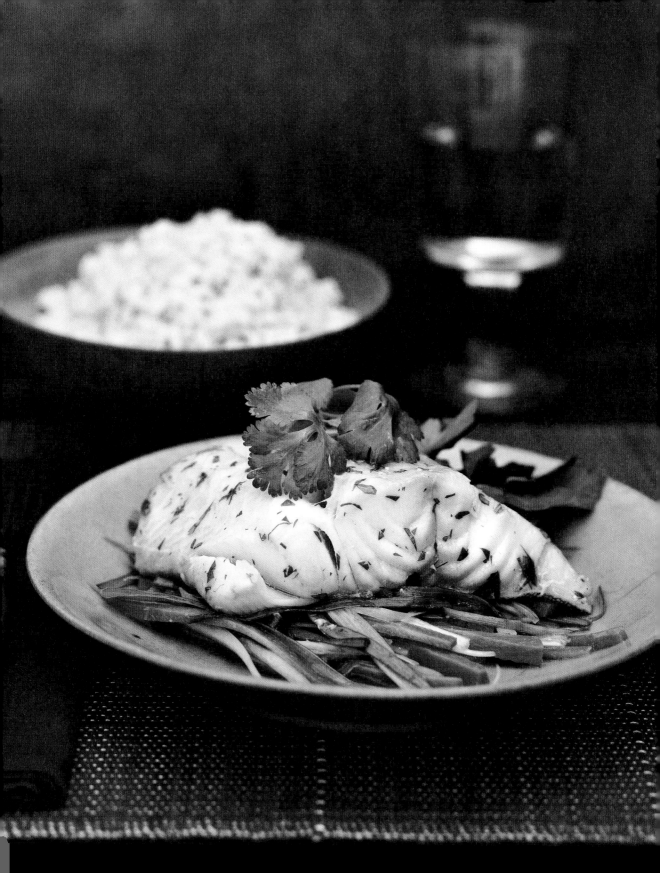

NUT-CRUSTED TILAPIA

PER SERVING:

417 CAL

38 g protein	
19 g carbohydrates	
3 g fiber	
26 g fat	
3 g saturated fat	
85 mg cholesterol	
262 mg sodium	

MAKES 4 SERVINGS

- 1 cup pecans
- 4 tilapia fillets (about 1½ pounds)
  - Salt
  - Freshly ground black pepper
- 3 tablespoons all-purpose flour
- 2 tablespoons 1% milk
- 1 tablespoon canola oil
  - Juice of ½ lime
- 1 cup salsa

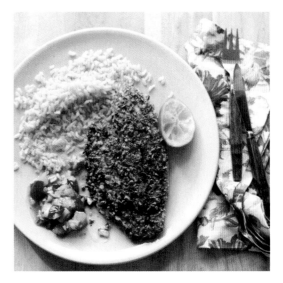

1. Finely chop the pecans in a food processor or put in a zip-top bag and crush with a mallet.
2. Season both sides of the fish with the salt and pepper.
3. Place the flour in a shallow bowl. Place the milk in another shallow bowl. Dredge the fish in the flour, shake off the excess, dip in the milk, and then coat thoroughly with the nuts.
4. Heat the oil in a large nonstick skillet over medium-high heat. Cook the fish for about 5 minutes in all, or until just done, turning once.
5. Stir the lime juice into the salsa in a small bowl and serve with the fish.

GRILLED SALMON

6   salmon fillets (4 ounces each and about 1$\frac{1}{2}$" thick), skin removed

$\frac{1}{2}$ teaspoon salt

$\frac{1}{4}$ teaspoon freshly ground black pepper

1.   Heat the broiler (or heat the grill to medium). Lightly coat the fish on both sides with cooking spray and sprinkle with the salt and pepper.

2.   Place the fillets on a baking sheet. Slide the sheet into the broiler about 4" from the heat and cook for 3 minutes. Flip the fish and continue cooking for 1 to 2 minutes longer, or until just done. (If grilling, place the fillets about 6" from the heat source.)

PER SERVING:

208 CAL

23 g protein

0 g carbohydrates

0 g fiber

12 g fat

2.5 g saturated fat

67 mg cholesterol

261 mg sodium

MUSTARD-AND-BROWN SUGAR-RUBBED SALMON

MAKES 4 SERVINGS

2 tablespoons firmly packed dark brown sugar

1½ teaspoons salt

1 teaspoon freshly ground black pepper

½ teaspoon ground cumin

¼ teaspoon mustard powder

4 salmon fillets (6 ounces each), skin removed

1 teaspoon olive oil

1. Stir together the sugar, salt, pepper, cumin, and mustard in a small bowl. Unwrap the fish and leave it on the paper you bought it in, placing it so the side that had skin is down. Press the sugar mixture evenly onto the fish.

2. Heat the oil in a large nonstick or cast-iron skillet over medium heat. When hot, place the fish rub side down in the pan. Cook for about 4 minutes, or until the rub dissolves and darkens slightly (being careful not to burn). Flip the fish and cook for about 1 minute, or to medium doneness.

Leftovers? If you made extra salmon, turn it into a dynamite salad: Just flake the salmon and toss it with a little oil and lemon or lime juice. Or stir the flaked fish into a rice, potato, or pasta salad.

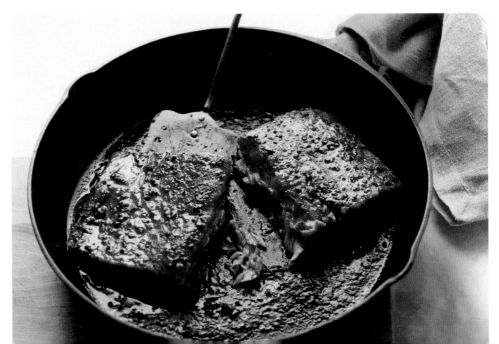

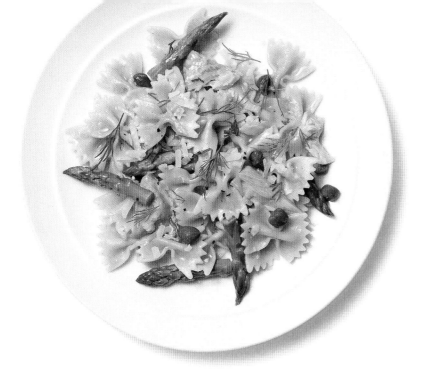

LEMONY SALMON-AND-DILL TOSS

MAKES 4 SERVINGS

- 1 can (7$\frac{1}{2}$ ounces) salmon, drained
- 1$\frac{1}{2}$ cups blanched asparagus pieces
- 3 tablespoons freshly squeezed lemon juice (from 1–2 lemons)
- 3 tablespoons chopped dill
- 2$\frac{1}{2}$ tablespoons olive oil
- 2 tablespoons capers
- 2 teaspoons lemon zest
- $\frac{1}{2}$ teaspoon salt
- $\frac{1}{2}$ teaspoon freshly ground black pepper
- 3 cups cooked farfalle
- $\frac{1}{3}$ cup shredded Parmesan cheese

PER SERVING:

342 CAL

22 g protein
35 g carbohydrates
3 g fiber
14 g fat
3 g saturated fat
48 mg cholesterol
736 mg sodium

Mix the salmon, asparagus, lemon juice, dill, oil, capers, lemon zest, salt, and pepper in a bowl. Stir in the farfalle and cheese.

GRILLED
SALMON BURGERS

PER SERVING:
170 CAL

23 g protein

1 g
carbohydrates

0 g fiber

7 g fat

1 g
saturated fat

60 mg
cholesterol

150 mg sodium

MAKES 4 SERVINGS

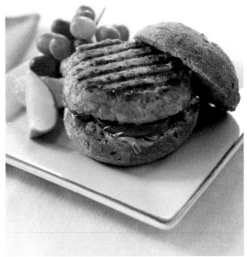

1 pound skinless salmon fillet (cut into 1" cubes)

1 tablespoon Dijon mustard

1 tablespoon grated lime zest

1 tablespoon peeled and minced fresh ginger

1 tablespoon chopped fresh cilantro

1 teaspoon reduced-sodium soy sauce

$\frac{1}{2}$ teaspoon ground coriander

Salt

Freshly ground black pepper

Fresh lime wedges

1. Preheat the grill to medium-high heat. Lightly coat the rack with olive oil cooking spray.

2. Pulse the salmon in a food processor, just enough to grind coarsely. Transfer to a large bowl and mix in the mustard, lime zest, ginger, cilantro, soy sauce, and coriander.

3. Form the salmon mixture into 4 patties and season with the salt and pepper to taste. Grill the burgers, turning once, for 4 minutes per side for medium, or until done. Garnish with the lime.

TUNA NOODLES WITH PEAS

MAKES 4 SERVINGS

PER SERVING:

528 CAL

28 g protein
53 g carbohydrates
6 g fiber
23 g fat
6 g saturated fat
82 mg cholesterol
987 mg sodium

1 large whole wheat pita or 2 slices whole wheat bread

8 ounces wide egg noodles

2 cups frozen peas

2 tablespoons olive oil

2 large cloves garlic, crushed

$\frac{1}{2}$ cup sour cream

2 cans (5 ounces each) tuna in olive oil, undrained

$\frac{1}{2}$ teaspoon salt

$\frac{1}{4}$ cup chopped flat-leaf parsley

Freshly ground black pepper

1. Pulse the pita or bread in a food processor until roughly chopped. Toast in a toaster oven for about 3 minutes, or until just golden brown. Set aside.
2. Cook the noodles according to the package directions, adding the peas during the last 2 minutes. Reserve $\frac{1}{4}$ cup of the cooking liquid and drain the noodles.
3. Add the oil and garlic to the pasta pot over low heat and cook for about 30 seconds, or until just beginning to color.
4. Turn off the heat. Stir in the reserved cooking liquid, sour cream, tuna (along with the oil), and salt and mix well. Stir in the pasta with the peas and parsley. Season to taste with the salt and pepper. Top with the reserved bread crumbs.

Save money: *Leftover bread going to waste? Make crumbs, as directed in step 1, above. They'll be cheaper and better than store-bought, and they'll keep in the freezer for months.*

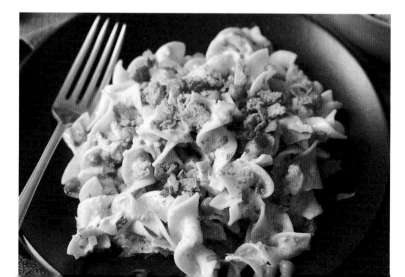

DESSERTS

HEAVENLY TIRAMISU

MAKES 9 SERVINGS

- 1 cup fat-free ricotta
- 8 ounces mascarpone (about ³⁄₄ cup)
- 2 tablespoons 2% milk or water
- 1 teaspoon vanilla extract
- ¹⁄₄ cup + 2 tablespoons sugar
- 1¹⁄₂ cups brewed espresso or 4 teaspoons instant espresso powder dissolved in 1¹⁄₂ cups boiling water
- 24 store-bought crisp ladyfingers (such as Savoiardi), 7 ounces total
- 2 teaspoons unsweetened cocoa powder

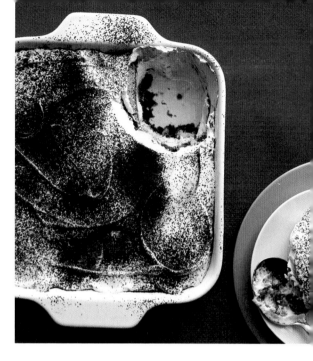

1. Put the ricotta, mascarpone, milk or water, vanilla extract, and ¹⁄₄ cup of the sugar in a food processor and process until creamy.
2. Combine the hot espresso and remaining 2 tablespoons sugar in a pie plate or shallow dish and stir until the sugar dissolves.
3. Dip each ladyfinger in the espresso mixture, working quickly, and arrange half of them in a single layer in an 8″ × 8″ baking or serving dish. Spread half of the ricotta mixture evenly on top. Put 1 teaspoon of the cocoa powder in a small strainer and dust over the cream. Repeat with the remaining ladyfingers, ricotta mixture, and 1 teaspoon cocoa powder.
4. Cover with plastic wrap and refrigerate for 6 hours or overnight before serving.

PER SERVING:
250 CAL

6 g protein
28 g carbohydrates
1 g fiber
12.5 g fat
6.5 g saturated fat
59 mg cholesterol
83 mg sodium

IRRESISTIBLE BROWNIES

PER SERVING:
305 CAL

| 5 g protein |
| 31 g carbohydrates |
| 2 g fiber |
| 22 g fat |
| 2 g saturated fat |
| 26 mg cholesterol |
| 73 mg sodium |

MAKES 8 BROWNIES

1/2 cup all-purpose flour

1/3 cup unsweetened cocoa powder, sifted if lumpy

1/4 teaspoon baking powder

1/8 teaspoon salt

2/3 cup firmly packed dark brown sugar

1/4 cup canola oil

1 large egg

1 large egg white

1 teaspoon vanilla extract

1/4 cup mini semisweet chocolate chips

1 cup chopped walnuts

1. Preheat the oven to 350°F. Coat an 8″× 8″ or 9″× 9″ baking pan with cooking spray.
2. Combine the flour, cocoa powder, baking powder, and salt in a large bowl.
3. Put the sugar, oil, egg, egg white, and vanilla extract in a small bowl. Whisk until smooth. Pour into the flour mixture and stir until blended. Stir in the chocolate chips and walnuts. (The batter will be stiff.)
4. Spread the batter in the prepared pan. Bake for 20 to 22 minutes, or until firm at edges and a wooden pick inserted off-center comes out with a few moist crumbs. Place the pan on a rack and let cool completely.

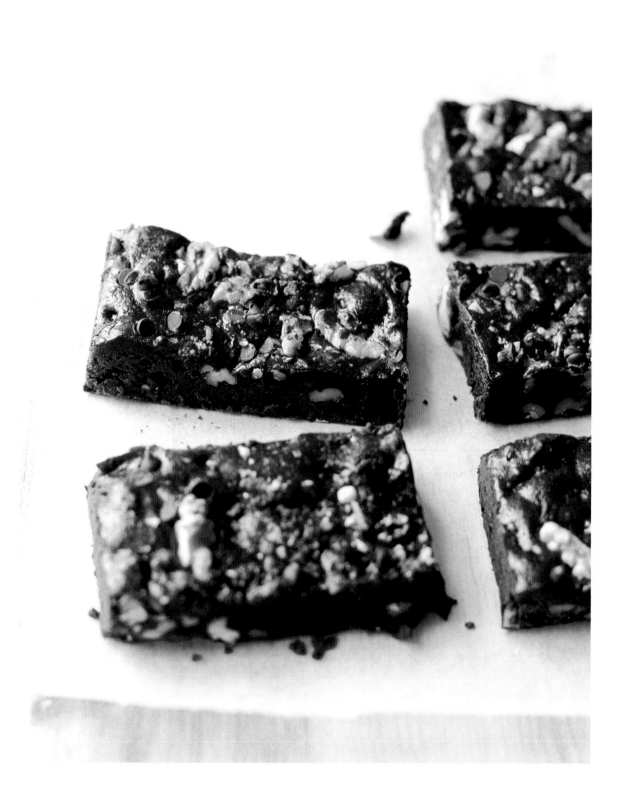

PB&C OATMEAL SNACK

PER SERVING:

267 CAL

9 g protein	
29 g carbohydrates	
4 g fiber	
14 g fat	
4 g saturated fat	
0 mg cholesterol	
134 mg sodium	

MAKES 1 SERVING

¼ cup quick-cooking oats

½ cup light vanilla soy milk

 1 tablespoon creamy peanut butter

 1 tablespoon mini semisweet chocolate chips

Stir together the oats and milk in a microwaveable bowl and microwave on high power at 30-second intervals, stirring in between, until the oatmeal reaches your desired consistency. Stir in the peanut butter and chocolate chips.

RICH CHOCOLATE TORTE

MAKES 16 SERVINGS

 1 tablespoon + ¼ cup cocoa powder
 1 cup walnuts
 ¾ cup sugar
 5 enriched eggs, separated
 ½ teaspoon cream of tartar
 ½ cup reduced-fat sour cream
 5 ounces bittersweet chocolate (60% cacao or higher), melted
 1 teaspoon ground cinnamon

1. Preheat the oven to 350°F. Coat an 8" or 9" springform pan with cooking spray and dust with 1 tablespoon of the cocoa powder.
2. Combine the walnuts and ¼ cup of the sugar in a blender or food processor. Pulse until finely ground. Set aside.
3. Beat the egg whites and cream of tartar in a large bowl with an electric mixer on high until foamy. Gradually add the remaining ½ cup sugar, beating, until stiff peaks form.
4. With the same beaters, beat the egg yolks in another bowl until thick. Add the sour cream, melted chocolate, cinnamon, and remaining ¼ cup cocoa powder and beat to blend well. Fold in the walnut mixture. Stir one-quarter of the egg whites into the chocolate mixture. Fold in the remaining whites in 2 batches.
5. Pour into the pan and bake for 45 minutes, or until a knife inserted in the center comes out clean. Cool the cake completely in the pan on a rack for at least 4 hours. (The cake is best made a day ahead and stored covered in the pan until serving.) Release the sides of the pan.

PER SERVING:

159 CAL

| 4 g protein |
| 17 g carbohydrates |
| 2 g fiber |
| 10 g fat |
| 3 g saturated fat |
| 59 mg cholesterol |
| 25 mg sodium |

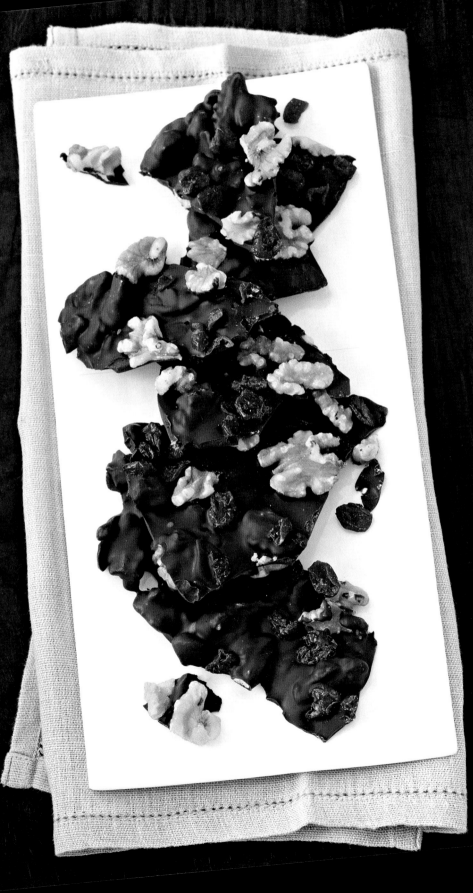

FRUIT 'N' NUT BARK

MAKES 8 SERVINGS

½ cup (60% cacao) chocolate baking chips
½ cup chopped walnuts
¼ cup dried cranberries

1. Line a baking sheet with parchment or waxed paper.
2. Place the baking chips in a medium bowl and microwave on medium power for 2 minutes, stirring twice, or until just melted. Stir in the walnuts and cranberries.
3. Spread the mixture on the baking sheet to form a 10" × 8" rectangle. Refrigerate for 1 hour, or until set. Cut or break the bark into 8 pieces.

PER SERVING:
109 CAL

2 g protein	
11 g carbohydrates	
1 g fiber	
8 g fat	
2 g saturated fat	
0 mg cholesterol	
1 mg sodium	

MAPLE-WALNUT BITES

MAKES 36 COOKIES (9 PER SERVING)

2 egg whites, at room temperature
¼ teaspoon cream of tartar
¼ cup maple sugar
½ cup walnuts, toasted and chopped

1. Preheat the oven to 250°F. Line 2 large baking sheets with parchment paper.
2. Beat the egg whites and cream of tartar in a large mixing bowl with an electric mixer on high speed until soft peaks form. Continue beating while gradually adding the maple sugar until very stiff and glossy peaks form. Gently fold in the walnuts.
3. Drop by tablespoons onto the parchment paper. Bake for 1 hour. Turn off the oven and leave in the oven for 1 hour without opening the oven door.

PER SERVING:
122 CAL

4 g protein	
10 g carbohydrates	
1 g fiber	
8 g fat	
<1 g saturated fat	
0 mg cholesterol	
29 mg sodium	

Note: *You can purchase maple sugar in health food stores as well as in many supermarkets.*

PEANUT BUTTER-AND-CHOCOLATE CHIP BARS

MAKES 16 BARS

- $^3/_4$ cup white whole wheat flour (such as King Arthur) or whole wheat pastry flour
- $^3/_4$ teaspoon baking soda
- Pinch of salt
- 1 cup enriched peanut butter
- $^1/_3$ cup Splenda Brown Sugar Blend
- 1 egg, beaten
- $^1/_2$ cup fat-free milk
- 1 teaspoon vanilla extract
- $^1/_2$ cup bittersweet chocolate chips

1. Preheat the oven to 350°F. Coat an 8″ × 8″ baking dish with cooking spray.
2. Combine the flour, baking soda, and salt on a large sheet of waxed paper. Stir with a fork.
3. Combine the peanut butter, brown sugar blend, and egg in a mixing bowl. Stir vigorously until creamy. Add the milk and vanilla extract. Stir until smooth. Add the flour mixture, stirring until well combined. Stir in the chocolate chips.
4. Spread the dough into the baking dish and pat the top to smooth. Bake for about 15 minutes, or until slightly puffy and very lightly browned at the edges. Remove and allow to cool for at least 10 minutes before cutting. Store at room temperature, tightly covered with foil.

LINZER THUMBPRINT COOKIES

MAKES 4½ DOZEN COOKIES

¾ cups slivered almonds

1 cup all-purpose flour

¼ cup whole wheat flour

1 teaspoon ground cinnamon

¼ teaspoon salt

½ cup firmly packed light brown sugar

¼ cup + 1 tablespoon unsalted butter

3 tablespoons 50/50 butter-blend spread (we used Smart Balance)

½ teaspoon almond extract

5 tablespoons raspberry 100% fruit spread

1 tablespoon confectioners' sugar (optional)

PER COOKIE:

46 CAL

1 g protein	
5 g carbohydrates	
0.5 g fiber	
2.5 g fat	
1 g saturated fat	
3 mg cholesterol	
12 mg sodium	

1. Preheat the oven to 350°F. Toast the almonds on a baking sheet for 10 minutes, or until light golden. Cool.
2. Whisk the flours, cinnamon, and salt in a bowl.
3. Grind the almonds in a nut grinder or pulse in a mini food processor with ⅓ cup of the dry mixture until finely ground. Whisk the almonds into the remaining dry mixture.
4. Beat the brown sugar, butter, spread, and almond extract in a medium bowl with an electric mixer on medium speed until combined. Add the dry mixture in thirds, beating to combine.
5. Shape the dough into disks, using 1½ teaspoons of dough for each. Place the cookies 1½" apart on ungreased baking sheets. Press the middle of each cookie with your thumb, reshape the dough if the edges split, and fill each indentation with a rounded ¼ teaspoon of the fruit spread.
6. Bake the cookies for about 10 minutes, or until the edges are golden. Cool to room temperature. Sift the confectioners' sugar over the cookies, if desired.

CINNAMON-PECAN DIAMONDS

MAKES 3 DOZEN COOKIES

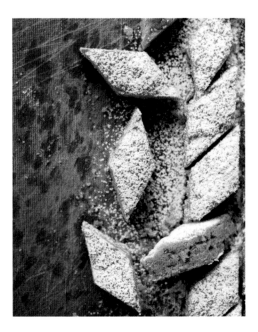

1	cup pecan pieces
1½	cups all-purpose flour
½	cup whole wheat flour
1	teaspoon ground cinnamon
¼	teaspoon salt
½	cup granulated sugar
½	cup unsalted butter
¼	cup 50/50 butter-blend spread (we used Smart Balance)
1	teaspoon vanilla extract
2	tablespoons confectioners' sugar

1. Preheat the oven to 350°F. Line a 9″ × 9″ baking pan with foil. On the baking sheet, toast the pecans for about 10 minutes, or until fragrant. Cool.
2. Whisk the flours, cinnamon, and salt in a bowl. Chop the pecans in a mini food processor with ⅓ cup of the flour mixture. Whisk back into the remaining flour mixture.
3. Beat the granulated sugar, butter, spread, and vanilla extract in a medium bowl with an electric mixer on medium speed until combined. Add the nut-and-flour mixture in thirds, beating on medium speed until combined.
4. Pat the dough evenly into the prepared pan. Transfer the foil and dough to the baking sheet. Cut the dough crosswise into 8 strips. Cut the dough on the diagonal into 10 strips. (The outside strips will be corners that don't make full cookies.). Bake for 25 minutes, or until the edges are golden brown.
5. Cut the cookies along the original score lines. Cool. Sift the confectioners' sugar over the cookies.

PHOTO CREDITS

©Masterfile: page vi (left), 95, 143, 146

©Getty Images: pages vi (right), viii (right), 2 (left), 2 (right), 9, 19, 20, 31, 46 (left), 53, 88 (center), 96, 131, 138 (left and center), 172 (right), 189, 202 (left), 209, 216, 218 (top right & bottom–2)

©Photodisc: pages vii (left), 101,

©Alexa Miller: pages vii (right), 150, 151

©Stockbyte: pages viii (left), 194,

©Kana Okada: pages ix (left), 241, 277, 278, 296, 299, 334, 350

©Alexandra Rowley: pages ix (right), 318

©BananaStock: page 2 (center), 218 (top left)

©Dan Winters: page 37

©Jonathan Kantor: page 46 (center), 119

©Kang Kim: page 46 (right), 159 (right), 287, 305, 308, 321, 341

©Levi Brown: pages 66, 69

©Jamie Chung: page 75

©Holly Lindem: page 82

©Thomas MacDonald: page 88 (left)

©Marcus Nilsson: page 88 (right), 231, 243, 246, 265, 267, 309

©Christa Renee: pages 105-111, 162, 167–169

©Dirk Anschütz: page 114

©Jonathan Pozniak: pages 123-126, 158, 159 (left), 160

©Photolibrary: page 134, 217

©Trunk Archive: page 138 (right)

©Kate Powers: page 172 (left)

©Veer: page 172 (center)

©Deborah Jaffe: page 178

©Geoffrey Sokol: page 184

©ItStock: page 186

©Juicy Images: page 197

©Folio-ID: page 202 (center)

©Age Fotostock: page 202 (right)

©Burcu Avsar: page 206

©Stephanie Rausser: page 212

©Plamen Petkov: page 222

©Con Poulos: page 234, 249, 255, 258, 275, 284, 291, 293, 303, 315, 325, 338, 340, 345, 347, 354

©John Kernick: page 250, 253, 261, 310, 343

©Mitch Mandel: page 272, 333, 342

©Hallie Burton: page 300, 317

©Yunhee Kim: page 304

©Mikkel Vang: page 307, 316, 327, 329

©David Prince: page 313, 337

©Charles Masters: page 320

©Sang An: page 330

INDEX

Underscored page references indicate boxed text or tables.

metabolic syndrome, treating with, 14
small, recommendations for, 130–35
Lifestyle factors in type 2 diabetes
genetics *versus,* 98
overview, 8
Lifestyle habits, establishing, 60
Lift and reach exercises, 79
Light trans-free margarine, 68
Linalool, 175
Listeria, 63
"Lite" meals, dodging, 89
London Broil
Bronzed London Broil, 313
Lower-body muscles, strengthening, 147
Low-fat creamy salad dressing, 72
Low-fat dairy products, 77
Low-fat yogurt, 68
Lp-PLA2, measuring, 75–76
Lunch
anti-bloat diet, 127
brown-bag, 134
cravings, quelling strategies, 90
exercise during lunch break, 140, 143
Summer-Body Diet, 112
Lunesta, 23
Lung cancer death risks, reducing, 207
Lung function, improving, 207

M

Macaroni
Macaroni and Cheese, 293
Macular degeneration risk, reducing, 144
Magnesium
breakfast as source of, 116
supplements, 24
Mail order medicines, 3
Making something, happiness, boosting by, 199
Margarine, 68
Marjoram, 50
Massage, 181–82
Maxalt, 24
Meal plans, 59
Meat
selection guidelines, 66–67
substitutes, 91
Meatballs
Mini Meatball Soup, 269

Meatloaf
Meat Loaf with Mushroom Gravy, 314–15
Medication. *See* Drugs; *specific* medication type
Meditation, 178–79
Mediterranean diet, 74, 225
Melanomas
as endometriosis shadow disease, 27–28
diabetes and, 28
Memory boosting
alliterations, creating, 203
cortisol role, 179
yoga techniques, 191
Menstrual cramps, 175
Metabolic disease risk factors, 89
Metabolic syndrome
as diabetes risk factor, 15
as heart attack and stroke risk factor, 13
indicators, 15, 26
kidney stones as shadow disease of, 26–27
overview, 14
risks
lowering, diet role in, 48, 74
visceral fat, 95
Metabolism, aging effect on, 162
Metformin (Glucophage), 18–19
Methotrexate, 22
Migraines
shadow diseases, 26, 27
treatment, 23–24
triggers, 174
MigreLief, 24
Milk, 67–68
Mindfulness (relaxation technique), 181
Minerals
as supplements, 59
foods fortified with, 60
Minirelaxation sessions, 175
Mirtazapine (Remeron), 21
Money-spending
giving money away, 198
happiness and, 173–74
Mood, boosting, rapid thinking role in, 174
Motion sickness remedies, 63
Motrin, 22, 24
Mountain Climber, 110
Muffins
Avocado Breakfast Muffin, 237
Multivitamins, 59